Self Assessment and Review of Dermatology

Self Assessment and Review of Dermatology

Vijay K Garg
MD, MNAMS, MAMS (Vienna)
Professor and Head
Department of Dermatology and STD
Maulana Azad Medical College
and
Lok Nayak, GNEC and GB Pant Hospital
New Delhi-110 002

Atul M Kochhar
MD, DNB, MNAMS
Specialist
Department of Dermatology and STD
Maulana Azad Medical College
and
Lok Nayak, GNEC and GB Pant Hospital
New Delhi-110 002

Kabir Sardana
MD, DNB, MNAMS
Assistant Professor
Department of Dermatology and STD
Maulana Azad Medical College
and
Lok Nayak, GNEC and GB Pant Hospital
New Delhi-110 002

PEEPEE
PUBLISHERS AND DISTRIBUTORS (P) LTD.

Self Assessment and **Review of Dermatology**

Published by
Pawaninder P. Vij

Peepee Publishers and Distributors (P) Ltd.
Head Office: 160, Shakti Vihar, Pitam Pura, Delhi-110 034 (India)

Corporate Office: 7/31, Ansari Road, Daryaganj, Post Box-7243
New Delhi-110002 (India)

Ph: 65195868, 23246245, 9811156083

e-mail: peepee160@yahoo.co.in

e-mail: peepee160@rediffmail.com

e-mail: peepee160@gmail.com

www.peepeepub.com

First Edition: **2006**

ISBN: 81-88867-95-0

Printed at: Lordson, C-5/19, Rana Pratap Bagh, Delhi-110 007

To…

… Our Parents to whom we all owe so much

and

… Our wives who tolerated our involvement in academic pursuit at the cost of family life

and

… Our children who due to our constant absence tolerated us at the cost of almost forgetting us

and

… All our students

and

… The motto of Bhagwad Gita

"Karamdharma"

"Tireless pursuit in your assigned task without any attachment to the consequence of action—good or bad"

PREFACE

Not only is dermatology a much sought after branch the world over, the potential for growth both academic and in practice has made this a very lucrative branch. In spite of all this, dermatology is not included in the final examination of MBBS.

But a knowledge of the subject is required in every PG entrance exam including AIPG, Delhi PG, AIIMS, CMC—Vellore, JIPMER, USMLE and PLAB. In view of the lack of extensive exposure of the subject in MBBS, a need for a brief, concise book targeted at tackling the MCQ based questions with a brief, succinct theory has long been felt.

Though the market is flooded with a number of books, many of them are not even framed by dermatology experts and lack correct and appropriate information. Also the authors of most books are not even conversant in teaching students.

At the end we have inserted the solved PG entrance exam papers of this year to enable the students to assess their knowledge. The suggestions and healthy critical remarks will very much be appreciated to improve this book.

Authors

ACKNOWLEDGEMENTS

We acknowledge the support, encouragement and patience of Mr. Pawaninder P Vij, Director M/s Peepee Publishers and Distributors Pvt. Ltd., whose persistence has been instrumental in taking out this book.

CONTENTS

Chapter 1

Basics of Dermatology

- Skin is the largest organ of the body covering an area of **$2m^2$** constituting **4 kg** of adult body weight.
- It is composed of:
  a. Epidermis.
  b. Dermis.
  c. Subcutaneous layer.
- Ratio of Epidermis to Dermis is 1 : 20.
- Layers of the **epidermis** from bottom to top.
- Basal cell layer/Stratum germinativum.
- Prickle cell layer/Stratum malphighii.
  – Granular cell layer/Stratum granulosum.
  – Stratum corneum.
- **Stratum corneum** is a dead layer. Stratum malphighii takes 28 days for its generation from basal layer.
- Most of the mitotic activity takes place in stratum basale.
- **Stratum lucidum** is an extra layer seen only in palms and soles. (Present between stratum corneum and stratum granulosum).
- Cells found in the epidermis are: Keratinocytes, Melanocytes, Langerhan's cells, and Merkel cells.
- Stratum malphighii—living layer of the skin.
- Keratinocytes constitute 90% of epidermal cells. The stratum granulosum contain odland bodies or membrane coated granules. They produce the lipid layer.
- Keratinocyte contains **profilagrin**—make the cytoskeleton of the keratin **(defect in ichthyosis vulgaris).**
- Melanocytes are dendritic cells that arise from neural crest. They synthesize melanin and transfer it to epidermal keratinocytes. A single melanocyte supplies 36 keratinocytes.
- Langerhan's cells are dendritic cells originating from bone marrow. Seen in suprabasal layer of epidermis, they express HLA-DR and antigens CD_1, and CD_4 on their surfaces. They also have surface receptors for C_3 and F_C fragment of IgG and can secrete interleukin-1. They contain "Ber beck granules" (racquet shaped).
- Merkel cells migrate from neural crest. Most numerous on digital pads, lips, oral cavity, and hair follicles, they are involved in sensation. They act as mechanoreceptors and contain neurotransmitter materials.
- Grenz zone is a narrow clear zone between epidermis and dermis **(Diagnostic in leprosy).**
- Total epidermal turnover time is 28 days.
- **The Dermis** consists of connective tissue, amorphous ground substance composed of mucopolysaccharide, blood vessels, nerves, lymphatic and muscles.
- The connective tissue is composed mainly of collagen (75%) and also elastic or reticulin fibres.

Cells Found in the Dermis

Lymphocytes, histiocytes, fibroblasts and mast cells.

- **The subcutaneous layer** contains fat, sweat glands and blood vessels.

Functions of the Skin

- Acts as a physical barrier.
- Prevents excessive absorption or loss of water.
- Involved in temperature regulation.
- Perceives sensation such as pain, touch, temperature.
- Involved in immunological reactions.
- Melanin pigments protects against UVL.
- Synthesizes vitamin D in presence of sunlight.

The Sweat Glands

They are of two types:
1. Eccrine.
2. Apocrine.
   - **The Eccrine sweat** glands are present all over the skin, particularly the palms, but not in the mucosae. Situated in the dermis, they secrete a watery fluid containing chloride, lactic acid, fatty acids, urea, glycoproteins and mucopolysaccharides **(Syringoma–eccrine gland tumor).**
   - **The Apocrine sweat glands** are vestigial remnants of odoriferous gland of lower animals. They are large and their pores open into the hair follicles. Found in the axillae, anogenital areas, nipples, areolas, umbilicus and scalp. Their secretion is sterile initially but due to bacterial action, it gets decomposed causing unpleasant smell. The glands do not function until puberty.
   Modified apocrine glands are the wax producing cerumen glands in the ear and mammary glands. They produce a white secretion containing proteins and complex carbohydrates **(Fox-fordyces disease–apocrine gland tumor).**
   - **The sebaceous glands:** They occur all over the skin except palms and soles—but are most numerous on the scalp and face. They have no lumen and their secretion is due to decomposition of the cells (Holocrine). The secretion, called sebum consists of fatty acids, cholesterol esters, wax, wax esters and squalene and is discharged into the pilo-sebaceous follicle.
   - **Hair:** Each hair consists of a shaft of keratinized cells produced by the hair bulb deep in the dermis and projects through the skin from the hair follicle. The hair follicle is richly supplied by nerves and blood vessels and contains melanin.

   There are three types of hair:
   1. Lanugo→hair covering the foetus.
   2. Vellus→non-medullated short, fine downy hair.
   3. Terminal→medulated coarse hair seen on scalp, beard, eyebrows and pubic region **(laser only affects terminal hair).**

The growth cycle of hair consists of 3 phases:
1. **Anagen** on the growth phase, may last upto 3 years (scalp hair).
2. **Catagen** on the transitional phase; may last upto 3 weeks.
3. **Telogen** on the resting phase–may last upto 3 months.

The length of the hair depends on the rate of growth and the length of anagen phase (3-5 years on the scalp).

- Shed telogen hair has a depigmented 'club' which differentiates it from shed anagen hair.
- Most hair are in the anagen phase (90%).
- The growth rate of scalp hair is 0.35 mm/day.

Primary Skin Lesions

1. <u>Macule</u>: A flat (without elevation or depression) area of change of colour of skin < 2 cm in diameter.

2. Patch: Same as macule but size > 2 cm.
3. Papule: A solid, circumscribed, raised palpable lesion measuring < 0.5 cm.
4. Plaque: A well circumscribed raised area of skin measuring > 0.5 cm in diameter can result from coalescence of papules. It can be raised or depressed **(morphoea).**
5. Nodule: A circumscribed, deeper, solid raised lesion of skin.
6. Vesicle: A fluid filled lesion (blister) < 0.5 cm in size.
7. Bulla: A fluid filled lesion > 0.5 in size.
8. Wheal: Well-defined, transient, raised, erythematous, itchy area of skin can vary in size.

SECONDARY LESIONS OF SKIN

1. Scales: Dried flakes of dead skin (keratin).
   - Sandpaper like scales founding → solar keratosis.
   - Silvery scales → psoriasis.
   - Greasy, yellow scale → seborrheic dermatitis.
   - Fine cigarette paper like scales → pityriasis rosea.
   - Limpet-like scales → Reiter's disease.
   - Yellowish brown scales → Darier.
   - Adherent scale (carpet-en-tack) sign–DLE.
2. Erosion: Superficial disruption of skin integrity (till papillary dermis).
3. Ulcer: Deep distribution of skin integrity (below papillary dermis).
4. Crust: Dried exudate on the skin.
5. Pustule: A pus-filled blister.
6. Atrophy: Thinning of skin.
7. Hypertrophy: Thickening of skin.

Some Important Terms used Dermatology

1. Excoriation: Linear erosions due to scratching **(only till basal layer commonly till stratum corneum).**
2. Erythema: Redness.
3. Erythroderma: Widespread redness and scaling of skin involving > 90% of body surface area. Can be due to numerous under lying causes e.g.: Psoriasis, seborrheic dermatitis, Pemphigus foliaceous or can be idiopathic.
4. Lichen is aggregation of small flat topped papules.
5. Lichenification: Thickening and hyper pigmentation of skin with exaggerated skin markings.
6. Milia: A small white papule filled with keratin.
7. Telangiectasia: A visible small dilated vessel on the skin.
8. Purpura: Pinpoint (1-2 mm) extravasation of blood into the skin, does not blanch on pressure.
9. Ecchymoses: Bruises > 3 mm in diameter.
10. Petechia: Bruises < 3 mm in diameter.

Nails: Nail is a hard, translucent plate of keratin that grows from beneath the proximal nail fold. A fingernail takes about 6 months to replace itself (growth rate = 0.1 mm/day or 1 cm/3 months). Toe nails grow at the rate of 0.03 mm/days. The growth of nails is affected by disease and malnutrition.

MULTIPLE CHOICE QUESTIONS

1. Isomorphic response is seen in all *except*:
- A. DLE
- B. Lichen planus
- C. Psoriasis
- D. Pemphigus

2. Acantholysis is seen in all *except*:
- A. Pemphigus
- B. Pemphigoid
- C. Herpes simplex
- D. Vaccinia

3. Match the following:
- A. Stratum granulosum
- B. Malphigian layer
- C. Sweat glands
- D. Sebaceous glands
- 1. Melanin
- 2. Myoepithelial cells
- 3. Hair follicle
- 4. Keratohyalin-granules

4. A 24-year-old man developed multiple asymptomatic papules and nodules with central necrosis on the face, neck and arms since one year. His ESR was 65 mm, and Mantoux test was strongly positive:
- A. Srofuloderma
- B. Lupus vulgaris
- C. Papulonecrotic tuberculid
- D. Miliary tuberculosis

5. All of following cells are found in epidermis *except*:
- A. Keratinocytes
- B. Melanocytes
- C. Langerhans cells
- D. Merkel cells
- E. Mast cells

6. One melanocyte supplies:
- A. 10 keratinocytes
- B. 36 keratinocytes
- C. 45 keratinocytes
- D. 20 keratinocytes
- E. 25 keratinocytes

7. Huxley's and Henley's layer is a part of:
- A. Hair
- B. Nail
- C. Skin
- D. Sweat gland

8. Langer's lines are seen in:
- A. Lichen planus
- B. Atopic dermatitis
- C. Psoriasis
- D. Normal persons

9. A whitish crescent shaped zone just distal to proximal nail fold is termed as:
- A. Hypomychinm
- B. Lunula
- C. Nail matrix
- D. Nail led

10. The turnover time of normal stratum corneum is:
- A. 7 days
- B. 14 days
- C. 21 days
- D. 28 days

1 D 2 B 3 A(4),B(1) C(2),D(3) 4 C 5 E 6 B 7 A 8 D 9 B
10 B

11. Duration of anagen phase for human scalp hair:
A. 3 weeks
B. 3 years
C. 3 months
D. 1 year

12. Histologically, "flame figures" are typically seen in:
A. Reiter's syndrome
B. Well's syndrome
C. Parapsoriasis
D. Lapus vulgaris

13. The turnover rate of epidermal cells on the scalp in dandruff is:
A. Decreased
B. Normal
C. Increased
D. Of no significance
E. None of the above

14. Neoplastic dyskeratosis is encountered in all *except*:
A. Bowen's disease
B. Solar Keratosis
C. Squamous cell carcinoma
D. Darier's disease

15. All true of woods lamp *except*:
A. Emits wavelength of 365 nm
B. Hypopigmented areas appear lighter
C. Epidermal pigmentation is enhanced
D. Dermal pigmentation is enhanced

16. All are types of epidermal melanin pigments *except*:
A. Phaemelanin
B. Trichochromes
C. Eumelanin
D. Dopachrome

17. Berkeley's membrane is seen in:
A. Pemphigus
B. Psoriasis
C. Pityriasis rosea
D. Pemphigoid

18. Syringoma arises from:
A. Eccrine sweat duct
B. Apocrine sweat duct
C. Eccrine sweat gland
D. Apocrine sweat gland

19. Normal epidermal turnover time is:
A. 52-75 days
B. 14-28 days
C. 75-100 days
D. 8-10 days

20. Sebum is composed of all *except*:
A. Triglycerides
B. Glycogen
C. Wax esters
D. Cholesterol esters
E. Squalene

21. Sweating is effectively inhibited by:
A. Atropine
B. β-blocker
C. Frusemide
D. Neostigmine

22. Stratum lucidum is seen in:
A. Hair and nails
B. Palms and soles
C. Normal epidermis
D. Scalp

23. The best fixative for a skin specimen is:
A. 40% formalin
B. Buffered neutral formalin
C. Absolute alcohol
D. Normal saline

11 B 12 B 13 C 14 D 15 D 16 D 17 B 18 A 19 A 20 B 21 A
22 B 23 B

24. The anatomic region where a wound is most likely to heal with a keloidal scar:
A. Face
B. Ear
C. Presternal area
D. Genitalia

25. Rate of growth of toe nail is:
A. 0.1 mm daily
B. 0.03 mm daily
C. 0.04 mm daily
D. 0.02 mm daily

26. Dermographism occurs in:
A. Cholinergic urticaria
B. Physical urticaria
C. Pressure urticaria
D. Urticaria pigmentosa

27. Cardinal sign of eczema is:
A. Papule
B. Macule
C. Erythema and itching
D. Vesicle

28. Treatment of choice for systemic candidiasis is:
A. Penicillin
B. Miconazole
C. Amphotericin
D. Nystatin

29. Duration of telogen phase for human scalp hair is:
A. 3 weeks B. 3 months
C. 3 years D. 1 year

30. Melanin synthesis is inhibited by:
A. Vitamin C
B. Oxidizing agents
C. Sulfhydryl containing compounds
D. Hydroquinone

31. Spectrum of UVA light is:
A. 200-290 nm B. 290-320 nm
C. 320-400 nm D. 400-700 nm

32. Wavelength of Wood's lamp:
A. 256 nm B. 365 nm
C. 300 nm D. 400 nm

33. Pitting of nails is seen in all *except*:
A. Psoriasis
B. Alopecia areata
C. Eczema
D. Lichen nitidus

34. Twenty-nail dystrophy seen in all *except*:
A. Alopecia areata
B. Lichen planus
C. Idiopathic
D. Psoriasis vulgaris

35. Birbeck granules are part of:
A. Langerhans cells
B. Keratinocytes
C. Melanocytes
D. Merkel cells

36. On electron menceoscopy melanocyte is readily distinguished from keratinocyte by:
A. Lack of desmosomes and tonofibrilis
B. Dendritic processes
C. Lack of golgi apparatus
D. Melanin content in the cyloplasm

37. Sutton's naevus is usually a benign melanocytic naevus but may be a:
A. Neuroid naevus
B. Blue naevus
C. Neuro fibroma
D. Primary or secondary malignant melanoma
E. All of the above

24 C 25 B 26 B 27 D 28 C 29 B 30 D 31 C 32 B 33 D 34 D
35 A 36 A 37 E

38. Cell detachment leading to acantholysis in Darier's disease is due to:
A. Autoantibodies directed against desmosomal components
B. Proteolysis of desmosomal proteins
C. Intercellular oedema
D. Intracellular oedema

39. Select the type of compress that one would employ for impetigo contagiso:
A. Normal saline compresses
B. Hypertonic saline compresses
C. Potassium permanganate compresses
D. Liquos pisis carbonis compresses

40. The correct concentration of potassium hydroxide for demonstrating the dermatophyte is:
A. 0.5%
B. 2%
C. 5%
D. 10%

41. Human mast cells produce the following mediators *except*:
A. Histamine
B. 5-hydroxytryptamine
C. Eosinophil chemotactic
D. Hyaluronic acid

38 B 39 C 40 D 41 B

Chapter 2

Infections and Infestations

COMMON INFESTATIONS OF THE SKIN

Scabies

- A common contagious skin disease caused by mite called sarcoptis scabieae hominis.
- Also called **seven-year itch.**
- Incubation period varies from 3-6 weeks.
- More common in **winters.**
- Predisposing factors → poor hygiene, overcrowding, low socio-economic group.
- Characterized clinically by severe nocturnal itching, usually positive family history and characteristic sites.
- Characteristic lesion is burrow which represents a tunnel made by female mite in stratum corneum (horny layer) in which to layer eggs. It measures 3-15 mm and ends in a small vesicle which contains the female mite.
- Other lesions are papules, vesicles, excoriations and crusted lesions.
- Typical sites → inter digital webs, front of wrist and forearm, elbows, axillae periareolar, periumblical areas, genitalia and buttocks, medial aspect of thighs, legs and feet.
- In infants face, scalp, neck, palms and soles may also be involved.
- **Life cycle** → After copulation female mite lays down 2-3 eggs/day in stratum corneum → eggs hatch to 6 legged larvae **(in about 1 week)** → converts into 8 legged adults (in about 2 weeks) (IMP: **topical therapy is repeated after one week**).
- Total time taken from egg to adult mite is 2-3 weeks.
- **Complications:**
  - Eczematization.
  - Secondary infection.
  - Urticaria.
    - Id eruption.
    - Lymphadenopathy.
    - **Glomerulonephiritis (due to nephritogenic strains of streptococci).**
    - Contact dermatitis to topical applications.

Variants of Scabies

1. Nodular scabies (mainly on genitalia).
2. Clean man scabies (only genital lesions).
3. Scabies incognito → seen in patients treated with steroids (topical).
4. Norwegian scabies → severe crusted variety seen in immunodeficient persons, old and debilitated persons, or malnourished individuals.

Treatment

ORAL: Ivermectol 200 microgram/kg dose repeated at one week.

1. Drug of choice is 5% permethrin cream (safe also in infants).
2. 1% gamma benzene hexachloride.
3. Crotamiton 10% (for children and infants).
4. 25% Benzyl benzoate (children 12.5%).
5. Sulphur ointment.
6. All family members should also be treated and clothes + bedclothes laundered.
7. Untreated cases last indefinitely.

IMP: **Safest topical drug Sulfur.**
Safest drug more than 3 months permethrin.
Contraindicated in pregnancy and infants -1% gamma benzene hexachloride.

Pediculosis

- Caused by lice, an oval, wingless 6 legged insect.
- It lays down several hundred eggs called Nits.
- Time taken in maturation i.e. from eggs to adult is 40 days.
- Intense itching is important symptom, which is due to the hypersensitivity to saliva injected at the time of biting or louse faeces.

Three types of Pediculosis are:

i. **Pediculosis Capitis** → caused by head louse.
  - Common site is back or side of scalp. **(Clinical presentation: Scalp pruritus with enlarged lymphadenopathy-mc presentation).**

ii. **Pedi. Corporis** → caused by body louse.
  - Lice does not reside on skin rather it resides on under clothing except when feeding.
  - Generalised itching all over the body is an important clinical feature.
  - **Vagabond disease** is caused by pediculosis corporis, in which there occurs pigmentation, excoriation, thickening and depigmented scar in a long standing case.

iii. **Pedi. Pubis** (also called pthirus pubis) → caused by crab louse.
  - Transmitted mainly by sexual contact.
  - Bluish or slate coloured macule is found, called Maculae-cerulea, which are found at side or trunk and inner aspect of thigh. **(Imp: Maculae-cerulea-faeces, altered blood).**

iv. **Pthirius palpebrum is eyelash involvement due to P. pubis.**
  - Other louse borne disease are Epidemic typhus fever, Relapsing fever and Trench fever.
  - **Drug of choice** in Pediculosis is **1%** Permethrin. Which kill both eggs and lice. 1% Gamma Benzene Hexachloride is more toxic and not ovicidal, hence it requires a second application after 1 week 0.5% malathion was used in the past.

Treatment of Pthirius palpebrum—Application of petrolatum or 1% physostigmine.

BACTERIAL INFECTIONS

Primary Pyodermas (Pyoderma arises in the normal skin).

- ***Impetigo:*** Two clinical patterns of impetigo are recognised: Bullous and non-bullous.
  a. Non-bullous (Impetigo contagiosa) is caused by either staphylococci or streptococcus pyogenes. The site of predeliction are the face and the extremities. It begins as a small, reddish macule which may soon turn into a vesicle. The vesicle has a thin roof that ruptures, leaving a raw, oozing area that quickly evolves into a yellowish crusted plaque **(honey colored crust).**
  b. Bullous impetigo: It is caused by staphylococci aureus phage group II. It occurs more commonly in the newborn and in older infants and is characterized by the rapid progression of vesicles to flaccid bullae occurring on a normal skin, containing clear yellow fluid that subsequently become dark yellow and turbid.

- ***Ecthyma***: Impetigo, if untreated, can extend more deeply producing shallow ulcer with black crusting. Ecthyma gangrenosum is a cutaneous ulcer caused by pseudomonas aeruginosa and resembles staphylococcal and streptococcal ecthyma. It occurs most commonly on the lower extremities of children or neglected elderly patients or individuals with diabetes mellitus.
- ***Folliculitis***: It is an infection of the hair follicle that may manifest either as superficial or deep folliculitis. Superficial folliculitis (impetigo of Bockhart) presents as a pinpoint to pinhead sized pustule at the follicular ostia. The sites of predilection include scalp and extremities. In deep folliculitis the infection extends deep in and around the hair follicle, the resulting perifolliculitis is responsible for marked inflammatory response. Sycosis barbae, furuncle, carbuncle, stye and perforating folliculitis of the nose are its morphological variants.
- ***Erysipelas and cellulitis***: Erysipelas present as a painful, bright red edematous indurated plaque with an advancing raised border, sharply demarcated from the surrounding normal skin. The legs and face are the most commonly involved sites. Cellulitis is a deep seated infection involving the subcutaneous tissue. The lesions in the cellulitis are not raised and no clear cut demarcation from uninvolved skin is seen and the constitutional symptoms are more pronounced.

Secondary pyodermas: Cutaneous lesions such as an abrasion, wound, eczematous lesion, fungul infection, ulcer and scabietic lesions may become secondarily infected.

Diagnosis: It is usually clinical but gram staining and culture of the exudate are helpful in the diagnosis.

Treatment: General measures: Improving the local hygiene, cleaning and removal of the bacteria laiden crusts and debris with potassium permanganate compresses.

Specific therapy: Topical therapy includes various topical antibiotics like mupirocin 2%, fusidic acid 1%, framycetin sulphate 1%. In patients with constitutional symptoms and widespread involvement, systemic therapy in the form of cephalosporins, macrolides, fluoroquinolines or cloxacillin are to be given.

MRSA—Drugs usually effective against MRSA are: Cloxacilin, Cepahlexin, Lincomycin, DOC-Linezolid, Mupirocin 2%, Vancomycin.

Tuberculosis of the Skin

Tuberculosis of the skin is caused by M. tuberculosis, M. Bovis and under certain circumstances, the bacillus calmette guerin (BCG) an attenuated strain of M. bovis.

Although mycobacterial diseases are widespread and serious, the organisms are neither very virulent nor very infectious, only about 5-10% of infections with M. tuberculosis lead to disease, the rate is similarly low for M. leprae and is very much lower for the facultative pathogens.

The two most frequent forms of cutaneous tuberculosis are lupus vulgaris and scrofuloderma. Generalised miliary tuberculosis is seen in infants (and adults with severe immunosuppression or AIDS) as is primary inoculation tuberculosis, scrofuloderma usually occurs in adolescents and the elderly, while lupus vulgaris may affect all age groups.

Classification of Cutaneous TB

Exogenous infection may occur as	1. TB chancre or Primary incoulation tuberculosis (i.e. infection of the non-immune host) 2. Tuberculosis verrucosa cutis (Infection of the immune host)
Endogenous spread may present	* 1 Lupus vulgaris **(mc form)** 2 Scrofuloderma (Mode of spread is contiguous **mc source is Lymph node**) * 3 Metastatic tuberculous abcess (tuberculous gumma)

* 4 Acute miliary tuberculosis
* 5 Orofacial tuberculosis (Mode of spread is Auto-inoculation)

Tuberculosis may occur rarely due to BCG Vaccination

Tuberculids - Lichen scrofulosorum
- Papulonecrotic tuberculid
- Facultative tuberculids
- Nodular vasculitis
- Erythema nodosum

1. ***Primary Inoculation Tuberculosis (Tuberculous Chancre, Tuberculous Primary Complex)***

Primary inoculation tuberculosis results from the inoculation of mycobacteria into the skin of a host not previously infected with tuberculosis. The tuberculous chancre and the affected regional lymph nodes constitute the tuberculous primary complex of the skin.

Most patients are children, but the lesions may also occur in adolescents and young adults, particularly in people working in professions related to medicine. All parts of the body may be affected, but sites of predilection are the face, hands and lower extremities which are readily injured. One third of the lesions are found on the mucous membranes of the conjunctiva and oral cavity.

Skin lesions occur as a result of entry into the skin via unnoticed abrasions, ritual circumcisions, infections with inadequately sterilised syringes, wounds, operations etc.

The tuberculous chancre initially present as a small papule, scab or wound with little tendency to heal. A painless ulcer develops, which may be insignificant or may enlarge to attain a diameter of over 5 cm. It is shallow with a granular or hemorrhagic base studied with miliary abscesses or covered by necrotic tissue. The ragged edges are undermined and of a reddish blue hue; as the lesions grow older, they become more indurated with thick adherent crusts.

Wounds inoculated with tubercle bacilli may heal temporarily but break down later, giving rise to granulating ulcers. Mucosal infections result in painless ulcers or fungating granulomas.

A slowly progressing, painless regional lymphadenopathy develops 3-8 wks after the infection and may rarely be the only clinical symptom. After weeks or months, cold abscesses may form which perforate to the surface of the skin and form sinuses. Fever, pain and inflammatory swelling of surrounding tissues simulating pyogenic infection are present in half the cases.

Histopathology: In early phase, there is an acute inflammation and mycobacteria are easily detected. After 3 to 6 weeks infiltrate and the regional lymph nodes acquire a tuberculoid appearance.

Differential Diagnosis: The differential diagnosis includes the primary complexes of syphilis, tularemia, sporotrichosis and ulcerative lesions of other mycobacterosis as well as other forms of skin tuberculosis.

Course: Without treatment, the condition may last upto 12 months lesions heal by scarring, in rare cases, lupus vulgaris occurs at the site of healed tuberculous chancre. In more than 50% of other cases the lymph nodes calcify.

Usually, the primary tuberculous complex yields satisfactory immunity, but reactivation of the disease may occur. Erythema, nodosum is a feature in 10% of the cases.

2. ***Tuberculosis verrucosa cutis (warty tuberculosis)***

This is a verrucous form of skin TB due to exogenous reinfection in previously sensitized individuals. Thus, tests with PPD (Mantoux) are highly positive. Inoculation of mycobacteria occurs at the sites of minor wounds or abrasions. Physicians, pathologists, medical students and laboratory attendants are at high risk due to infection from tuberculous patients or from autopsy material. Therefore, they are also called as **"Verruca necrogenica", "Anatomists wart", "postmortem warts" and "prosectors warts" (in pathologist).** **Lesions** usually occurs on the hands (most often on the radial border of the dorsum and on fingers). Lesions are asymptomatic and start as a small papule with purple inflammatory halo later they become hyperkeratolic and are often mistaken for a common wart slow growth and peripheral expansion lead to the development of a verrucous plaque with clefts and fissures discharging pus extending into the underlying infiltrated base.

Histopathology show ***psedoepithelio-matous hyperplasia*** with marked hyperkeratosis and dense inflammatory infiltrate. Abcesses form in the superficial dermis or within the pseudoepitheliomatous rate pegs. Epitheliod cells and giant cells are found in the mid dermis and beneath the epidermis.

Differential Diagnosis: Blastomycosis, Chromomycosis, and bromoderma be similar clinically and histopathologically.

Course: The evaluation of the lesions is slow and without treatment the course extends over many years secondary pyogenic infection may occur. Spontaneous involution does occur and usually results in sunken atrophic scans.

LUPUS VULGARIS

Lupus vulgaris is an extremely chronic and progressive form of tuberculosis of the skin occurring in individuals with moderate immunity and a high degree of tuberculin sensitivity.

Lupus vulgaris originates from tuberculosis elsewhere in the body by haematogenous, lymphatic, or contiguous spread most often from cervical adenitis or pulmonary tuberculosis, sometimes from an old, apparently quiescent primary complex.

Lesions are usually solitary; in patients with active pulmonary TB, multiple foci may develop.

In about 90% of the patients, the **head and neck** are involved. It usually starts on the nose or check and slowly extends onto adjacent areas.

In general, lupus vulgaris is asymptomatic. Initial lesion is a reddish brown macule or papule with soft, friable consistency. Upon diascopy, the infiltrate exhibits a **typical apple-jelly color**. Progression is characterized by an elevation of the lesions and a deeper brownish color. Involution in one area and expansion in another result in plaques with gyrate outline.

Various morphological variants of lupus vulargis have been described which include the plaque variety, papular, nodular, ulcerative, regetating and tumours like lesions.

Mucosal involvement may also occur nasal lesions start as nodules which ulcerate and may even destroy the cartilage.

Following a transient impairment of immunity, particularly after measles (post exanthematicus), multiple disseminated lesions may arise simultaenously in different regions of the body due to haematogenous spread from a latent tuberculosis focus.

Histopathology shows most importantly the formation of typical tubercles secondary changes may be superimposed. Epidermal thinning and atrophy or acanthosis with excessive hyperkeratosis or pseudoepitheliomatous hyperplasia. Differential lesions of lupus vulgaris should be differentiated from lesions of sarcoidosis, lymphocytoma, discoid lupus erythematosus, tertiary syphilis, leprosy, blastomycosis or other deep mycotic infections, lupoid leishmaniassis and chronic vegetating pyodermas.

Course: Lupus is extremely chronic. It is generally progressive and leads to considerable impairment of function and to disfiguration.

The most serious complication of long standing lupus is the development of carcinoma, mainly squamous cell type.

In 40% of patients with lupus there is associated tuberculous lymphadenitis, and 10 to 20 percent have pulmonary TB or TB of the bones and joints.

(*Clinical History:* Chronic, buttocks, anular, central scarring, children/young adults.)

Scrofuloderma

Scrofuloderma is a subcutaneous tuberculosis leading to cold abscess formation and a secondary breakdown of the overlying skin.

It results from contiguous involvement of the skin overlying another tuberculous process, most commonly tuberculous lymhadenitis tuberculosis of bones and joints, or tuberculous epididymitis. It may affect all age groups. The skin lesions first present as firm, subcutaneous nodules or as a well defined, freely movable asymptomatic infiltrate. The infiltrate enlarges and becomes doughy but it takes months before there is liquefaction with subsequent perforation, ulcers and sinuses develop. Ulcers are linear or serpingnous with undermined, inverted bluish edges and uneven, soft and granulating floors.

Histopathology shows massive necrosis and abscess formation in the center of the lesion. The periphery of the abscesses or the margins of the sinuses contain tuberculoid granulomas and true tubercles and M. tuberculosis can be found.

Differential Diagnosis: M. avium intracellulare and M. Scrofulaceum infection, syphilitic gumma, deep fungal infection particularly sporotrichosis, actinomycosis, severe forms of acne conglobata and hidradenitis suppurativa have to be excluded.

Course: Spontaneous healing does occur slowly leaving behind scar tissue. Lupus vulgaris may develop at the site of scrofuloderma or in its vicinity.

Metastatic Tuberculous Abscess (Tuberculous Gumma)

It occurs due to haematogenous spread of mycobacteria from a primary focus during a period of lowered resistance resulting in single or multiple cutaneous and subcutaneous lesion. It usually occurs in undernourished children of low socioeconomic status or in immunodeficient people, occasionally it may cause a carpal tunnel syndrome.

Ulcers and fistulaes may form over the abscesses. Metastatic tuberculous abscesses may occur with progressive organ tuberculosis or in miliary tuberculosis but may occur without any tuberculous focus also.

Histopathology shows massive necrosis and abscess formation usually copious amounts of mycobacteria are revealed.

All forms of panniculitis, deep fungal infections, syphilitic gumma and hidradenitis suppurativa have to be excluded.

ORIFICIAL TUBERCULOSIS (TUBERCULOSIS ULCEROSA CUTIS ET MUCOSAE)

Orificial TB is rare form of TB of the mucous membranes and the skin of the orifices due to autoinoculation of mycobacteria from progressive tuberculosis of internal organs, e.g., in intestinal or genitourinary TB.

In orificial TB of the mouth, the tongue is most frequently affected particularly the tip and the lateral margins. In advanced cases ulcers on lips along with ulcerative TB of larynx and pharynx may occur.

In intestinal TB, lesions develop on and around anus, and in females with active genitourinary disease, the vulva is involved. A small yellowish or reddish nodule appears on the mucosa and breaks down to form a circular or irregular ulcer with typical punched out appearance, undermined edges and soft consistency.

Histopathology shows massive non-specific inflammation, but tubercles with caseation may be found deep in the dermis. Mycobacteria are easily demonstrated.

Syphilitic lesions, aphthous ulcers and carcinoma have to be differentiated.

Orificial TB is a symptom of advanced internal disease with most unfavorable prognosis.

ACUTE MILIARY TUBERCULOSIS OF THE SKIN (Tuberculosis Cutis Miliaris Disseminata)

Miliary TB of the skin is an extremely rare skin manifestation of fulminating miliary TB due to haematogenous dissemination of mycobacteria. Tubercular sensitivity is usually absent Disseminated minute erythematous macules or papules occur all over the body, mainly on the trunk.

Histopathology shows inflammation and small abscesses and vasculitis. Mycobacteria are present both in and around blood vessels. In later stages/if patient develops immunity lymphocytic cuffing of vessels and even tubercles may be observed. Prognosis of this form is generally poor.

BCG Inoculation

Specific lesions following BCG vaccination include the following:

1. Lupus vulgaris may develop at or in the vicinity of the vaccination site after a latency of several months or years.
2. Individuals previously sensitive to tuberculin may exhibit a type of Koch's phenomenon. Regional adenitis along with general symptoms may be present.
3. Local subcutaneous abscesses may form.
4. Severe regional adenitis is the most common complication scrofuloderma may develop, and suppuration may persist for 6 to 12 months.
5. Generalised tuberculid like eruption may occur.
6. Generalised adenitis, osteitis, etc may also occur.
7. Fatal disease is rare—1 per 10 million vaccinated and occurs in immunocompromised.

Originally the tuberculids were considered to represent disseminated or systemic skin reactions to toxins of tubercle bagcilli, with a tendency to spontaneous involution. But, actually the evidence supporting the tuberculous etiology of tuberculids is largely circumstantial.

Tuberculids can be classified as:

Tuberculids (condition in which M. tuberculosis bovis).

Lichen serofulosorum, Papulonecrotic tuberculid.

Facultative tuberculids: Nodular vasculitis, erythema induratum, erythema nodosum.

Non tuberculids: Lupus miliaris disseminata faceii **(LMDF/acne agminata—variant of Rosacea).**

Lichen Scrofulosorum

It is lichenoid eruption of minute papules occurring in children and adolescents with tuberculosis.

It occurs due to a haematogenous spread of mycobacteria in an individual strongly sensitive to M. tuberculosis and is usually associated with chronic tuberculous disease of the lymph nodes and bones.

The eruption is asymptomatic, confined to the trunk and consists of small firm, follicular or para follicular papules having a flat top or bearing a minute horny spine or fine scales on their surface. Lichenoid grouping is pronounced and results in formation of rough, discoid plaques that tend to coalesce.

Histopathology shows superficial tuberculoid granulomas around hair follicles or independent of the adnexae. Mycobacteria are not seen and cannot be cultured from biopsy maternal.

Papulonecrotic Tubercluid: This is symmetric eruption of necrotising papules appearing in crops and healing with scar formation.

Disseminated crops of dusky red, symptomless, peasized papules appear mainly on the extension aspects of the extremities, buttocks and lower trunk. They may show a central depression and an adherent crust over a crater like ulcer. There in spontaneous involution resulting in pitted scars.

Histopathology shows a characteristic wedge shaped necrosis of the upper dermis extending into the epidermis. Involvement of the blood vessels is a cardinal feature and consists of obliterative or granulomatous vasculitis leading to thrombosis and complete occlusion of the vascular channels.

Eruptions due to pityriasis lichenoides et varioliformis acuta, lichen urticatus, prurigo and secondary syphilis form the differential diagnosis of papulonecrotic tuberculid.

Nodular Vasculitis (Erythema Induratum of Bazin)

It is a chronic sec recurring nodular and ulcerative disorder of the lower legs.

Patients of nodular vasculitis present with erythrocyanotic changes of lower extremities and heavy legs, with thick and firm but not edematous skin, and follicular perniosis.

(*Clinical points:* Female, thigh ulcerative nodules.)

Atypical Mycobacteria (Table 2.1)

i. **Rapid growers**—M. Fortuitium, cheloniae —Injection abscess.

ii. **Slow growers:**
- **Photochromogens**—marinum, kansasii–**Swimming pool granuloma.**
- **Scotochromogens**—Scrofulaceum, avium intercellulare complex.
- **Non-photochromogens.**
- (Second most common mycobacterial disease in the World–**M Ulcerans**—chronic leg ulcers).

FUNGAL INFECTIONS

Superficial Fungal

1. Dermatophytosis.
2. Candidiasis.
3. Pityriasis versicolor.
4. T. nigra and piedra.

Dermatophytosis

These are superficial fungal infections of the keratinized structures such as skin, hair and nails, caused mainly by the species of three genera of fungi, Trichophyton, Epidermophyton and Microsporum. The dermatophytosis infections are classified according to the anatomic area of involvement into various types.

Table 2.1: Summary of atypical mycobacterial infections

Organism	*Disease*	*Clinical Features*	*Treatment*
M. marinum	Swimming pool granuloma, fish tank granuloma feet	Warty plaque or sporotrichoid lesions on knees, elbows and Rifampin and ethambutol or tetracycline	
M. ulcerans	Buruli ulcer	Subcutaneous nodules rupture to form shallow ulcers with necrotic fat in the floor	Surgery is the treatment of choice followed by rifampin or cotrimoxazole
M. avium complex		Nodules, leg ulcers and papules Disseminated heterogenous infection in HIV patients	Combined therapy of isoniazid, rifampin and streptomycin
M. chelonae M. fortuitum	Injection abscess	Cellulitis and subcutaneous	Surgical debridement & amikacin or doxycycline or ciprofloxacin

Tinea capitis is a dermatophytosis of the scalp and associated hair that is caused by a variety of species of the genera microsporum and trichophyton.

- Ectothrix—Involves outside the hair shaft—Fluoresce green **(All except Trichophyton Tonsurans, violaceum).**

Types—Gray Patch, Seborrheic Type

- Endothrix—Invades the hair shaft—Do not fluoresce—**Trichophyton Tonsurans, violaceum** Black dot, agminate folliculitis.
- Tinea favosa or favus—**Trichophyton schoenlenii.**

Clinically an inflammatory or non-inflammatory alopecia occurs predominantly in children. It may present as grey patchy alopecia. The hair are broken at varying lengths and are dull grey in colour, due to the coating of the hair surface by arthrospores.

(*Imp:* Alopecia, scaling, itching—Wood's lamp—Tinea Capitis).

Black dot is a distinct entity recognized by the formation of relatively non-inflammatory alopecia. Hair breaks close to the scalp and appear as black dots. Scaling is minimal or absent. This variety of tinea capitis is most often caused by endothrix organisms such as T. tonsurans or T. violaceum.

Inflammatory type of tinea capitis is caused most commonly by zoophilic organisms. Clinically, a spectrum of inflammatory changes may be seen, ranging from a pustular folliculitis to a kerion, which present as an inflammatory, boggy mass shudded with broken hairs, oozing purulent material **(Kerion-KOH negative).**

Tinea favosa or favus is a chronic infection of the scalp characterized by the formation of yellowish crusts within the hair folicles (scutula) and eventuating in a cicatrizing alopecia.

Treatment: GRISEOFULVIN -10-20 mg/kg/day for 6-8 weeks or 2 weeks after clinical resolution.

T. barbae is a fungal infection of the beard and moustache area of the face with invasion of the coarse hair.

T. facie is the infection of the glabrous skin of the face and is commonly seen in the children.

T. corporis or T. circinata includes all dermatophyte infection of the glabrous skin with the exclusion of certain specific locations (i.e. palm, soles, groin). It presents as circinate lesion with central clearing and peripheral spreading inflammatory border or eczematous itchy plaques.

T. pedis or athlete's foot is the ring worm infection of the feet and may present as hyperkeratotic dry squamous inflammation of the soles and interdigital areas.

T. mannum is the fungal infection of the hand with morphology similar to T. pedis.

Tinea cruris also called Dhobi's itch is the intertrigenous infection localized to the groin, perineum and perineal region.

Tinea ungium or onychomycosis is the dermatophytic infection of the nail. It is recognized as:

i. Distal subungual omychomycosis in which the fungus invades the nail from the distal free edge **(Most common–Distal Lateral TYPE).**
ii. White superficial type which is characterized by the primary involvement of the surface of the nail plate that display small superficial white patches.
iii. Proximal subungual onychomycosis, characterized by the involvement of the nail plate from proximal nail fold **(Associated with HIV).**
iv. Total dystrophic onychomycosis in which the total destruction of the nail plate.
v. Endonyx **(rarest).**

Diagnosis of dermatophytosis is based on the clinical features, Wood's lamp examination, especially for T. capitis, microscopic examination of the skin scrapings or hair or nail clipping to demonstrate fungal hyphae or spores in 10-20% KOH solution, and culture in Sabouraud's agar medium.

Treatment may be topical or systemic depending upon the site, extent and severity of the infection. Various topical therapies includes: Azoles (e.g. 1% clotimuzole), allylamines (e.g. terbinfine), tolnaftate, ciclopirxolamine.

Systemic therapy includes griseofulvin (10 mg/kg/day),fluconazole, ketoconazole, tertbinafine, iatraconazole.

T. Versicolor or P. Versicolor

Pityriasis versicolor is a chronic recurrent non-inflammatory, superficial fungal infection of the skin caused by Malassezia furfur. The disease is seen as scaly, multiple hypo or hyper pigmented irregular macules most often occurring on the trunk and proximal extremities. The lesions are asymptomatic but few patients may complain of itching and/or mild burning. The lesions fluoresce **golden yellow** under the Wood's lamp.

(**Key points:** Chest, summers, mild scaling, usually white in color.)

Sign: Coup-de-ongle sign of Besnier- Increase scaling on scraping).

Diagnosis is mainly clinical. The organism can be readily identified in wet mounts of skin scrapings with 10% potassium hydroxide. **"Spaghetti and meat ball'** appearance of the yeast is quite characteristic.

Treatment includes 2.5% selenium sulfide washings, topical azole antifungus or oral treatment with ketoconazole, fluconazole, iatraconazole.

Candidiasis

Candidiasis is a superficial fungal infection that may involve almost any of the cutaneous and/or mucosal surface of the body. ***Candida albicans*** is most often associated with human infection. It is found as a commensal on the skin surface, oral cavity and gastrointestinal tract of healthy individuals, however under certain favourable condition it may become pathogenic.

Oral candidiasis or thrush presents as a sharply defined patch of creamy, curdy white, pseudomembrane which on removal reveal a raw erythematous area. The buccal mucosa, tongue, gums and palate are usually affected. In severe case it may extend to the esophagus and pharynx.

Perleche or angular cheilitis is characterized by erythema, soreness and fissuring at the angle of the mouth. Malnutrition, lip licking, excessive salivation, dental malformations may predispose to angular cheilitis.

Candidal intertrigo begins as erythematous bright red, scaly, flat topped papules in the folds and the edges are studded with pustular satellite lesions.

Candidal paronychia affects the proximal nail space which becomes red and swollen. There is loss of cuticle and the nail fold become detached from the nail plate, resulting in pocketing. Nail dystrophy with discoloration around the lateral nail fold develops in the later stages.

Therapy include topical or systemic antifungal agents like azoles (e.g. clotrimazole), nystatin terbinafine, ketoconazole; and systemic drugs such as fluconazole, iatraconazole.

VIRAL INFECTION

CHICKEN POX

I. Causative virus is Herpes zoster/Varicella zoster virus of B. subgroup of Herpes viruses.

II. Transmission is by droplets through naso-oral route. A patient is infectious **2 days before to 5 days** after the appearance of rash.

III. C/F usually affects children 2-10 years of an upper respiratory infection for a day or two followed by a morbilliform erythema leading to minute papules that within hours turn into vesicles of clear fluid. The fluid also turns purulent/turbid which then gets surrounded by a red coloured halo **(dew drop**

on a rose petal appearance).The vesicles and pustules persist for 2-4 days, get crusted, which finally separate to leave a shallow pink depression, healing without scarring. The lesions are polymorphic (i.e. different stages of lesions present together) and are centripetal in distribution, most numerous on the trunk, then face and limbs. Oral and conjunctival mucosa may also be involved.

IV. **Complications:** More common in immunocompromised adults. They are encephalitis, pneumonitis, hepatitis, arthritis, Reye's syndrome, secondary infection, symptomatic thrombocytopenic purpura, Stevens Johnson syndrome, keratitis. Infection during 1st 4 months of pregnancy can cause congenital malformations in the baby like micrognathia, eye defects, and encephalomyelitis.

V. **Diagnosis:** Tzanck smear from the base of a vesicle stained with giemsa shows giant cells and cells with inclusion bodies.
Direct immunofluorescence and PCR and complement fixation techniques can also be used.

VI. Rest and treatment of secondary infection. Antiviral therapy includes higher doses of Acyclovir (10 mg/kg 8 hourly I/V) usually 800 mg 5 times/day for 7-10 days. Others used are valaciclovir and famciclovir.
- The treatment should be started as soon as possible, preferably within 1st 48 hours to reduce the duration as well as complications of the disease.
- The disease confers life-long immunity.

Zoster (Shingles)

I. Causative organism same as of chickenpox.

II. Transmission by droplet as well as by direct contact.

III. C/F considered as a reactivation of a dormant virus after causing primary infection in the form of chicken pox. Fever and neurologic pain may precede the onset of groups of vesicles on an erythematous and edematous base situated unilaterally within the distribution of a cranial/spinal nerve.

The vesicles contain clear/purulent/hemorrhagic fluid and may ulcerate. The dermatomes most commonly affected are thoracic, cranial, lumbar and sacral. Severe hyperaesthesia and itching may persist through out the course of the disease. In 25% of cases, the lesions are followed by persistence of pain at the site, referred to as, post herpetic neuralgia which may last for years.

Herpes zoster ophthalmicus is the herpetic infection of the ophthalmic, periorbital and forehead skin. Vesicles may also form in the eye which then burst into ulcers, scarring and cause blindness.

Treatment same as of chicken pox. For post herpetic neuralgia—Bed rest with local heat, topical anesthetics have been advised. Also Tricyclic antidepressants and anti psychotics. Also I/V or oral acyclovir, systemic corticosterids. Strong analgesics have been advised (topical capsaicin).

INFECTIOUS MONONUCLEOSIS

I. Caused by Ebstein Barr virus, a Herpes virus of g-subgroup.

II. Transmission is by droplet infection through the respiratory route.

III. C/F Fever with B/L cervical adenopathy with pharyngitis, headache and malaise. The skin lesions are periorbital and there is lid edema with macular/morbiliform rash. Mucosal petechiae at the palate are seen.

IV. *Diagnosis*—Blood picture shows characteristic atypical lymphocytosis (**Downey cells**-abnormality large lymphocytes with fenestrated nuclei and foamy cytoplasm) and leukocytosis. Serology by positive heterophile aggulutination tests and IgM & IgG antibodies to virus are used.

V. *Treatment*—No specific treatment.

Ampicillin used for pharyngitis may give rise to generalised discrete itchy rash.

Bed rest with analgesics, saline gargles are helpful.

Other Herpes Viruses

HHV-6: Causes roseola infanticum/sixth disease Exanthema subitum.

HHV-7: Chronic fatigue syndrome and Roseola infantum.

HHV-8: Assoc. with Kaposi's sarcoma.

HPV

Human papilloma viruses belong to papovavirus group of DNA viruses that infect the squamous epithelia of human causing asymptomatic warty growths of the skin. To date, 77 types of HPV have been recorded.

WARTS (VERRUCAE) (Cutaneous Warts)

I. Transmission by Direct/Indirect contact, trauma, genital inoculation, swimming pools, meat handling or delivery through infected genital passage etc.

II. *Common warts (Verruca Vulgaris):* Caused mainly by **HPV-2 (also HPV 57, 1 and 4)** is an elevated rounded tumorous growth with a rough grey dry surface seen mostly over the back fingers, knees but can be present anywhere on the skin. Usually asymptomatic but those on palmar aspects of fingers and around nails can be painful. Other types of warts, depending on their site and morphology are:

Plantar warts present over the pressure points over the soles. Mainly caused **by HPV 1, 2 and 4.**

Plane warts (flat/V. plana) are multiple, 1-3 mm size, smooth, flat surfaced slightly raised, skin coloured papules caused mainly by **HPV 3 and 10.**

Filiform and digitate warts are usually, single, soft shrub like/finger shaped, thin projections seen over the scalp, fingers, face and neck.

Anogenital warts (**condyloma acuminatum**) are the warts present over the perianal and genital areas. These are spread mostly by sexual contact in sites of greatest friction. Caused mostly by **HPV 6 and 11.**

III. *Diagnosis*: Besides, the characteristic clinical appearance, the diagnosis can be confirmed on histopathology by presence of vacuolated cells called **koilocytes and inclusion bodies.**

IV. *Course:* The disease is usually benign with spread promoted by minor trauma like shaving and the lesions usually disappear within 1-2 years but HPV has been associated with many malignant and premalignant lesions as well, especially cervical dysplasia, Bowenoid papulosis, Buschke lowenstein disease, oral leukoplakia etc.

V. *Treatment:* The treatment includes both topical application and surgical methods.

Topical Treatment: Application of caustics (TCA, etc.), salicylates.

Podophyllin/podophyllotoxin, Gluteraldehyde, formalin, Retinoids etc.

Surgical treatment: Cryotherapy Electrodessication, Laser etc. Interferons.

I/L Bleomycin and topical 5-FU have also been used **(New drug: Imiquimod).**

MOLLUSCUM CONTAGIOSUM

It is a very common infection in children age 2-4 years and is spread through direct contact.

C/F: The infection comprises multiple, tiny (2-5 mm diameter) dome shaped, shiny translucent waxy papules with a **central umbilication.** The lesions have a tendency to spread/suppurate, to cause eczema, perilesional dermatitis, conjunctivitis etc. The lesions are common over face, hands and during sexual transmission over the anogenital region.

Diagnosis by histopathology showing **Molluscum or H.P. Bodies** which are eosinophilic intracytoplasmic inclusion bodies.

Best treated with currettage. Other modalities are diathermy cryotherapy, chemical cautery (TCA), topical retinoic acid/phenol/cantharidines.

(*Clinical Clue:* Child, Face, Umbilicated.)

Closest DD-Cryptococcus.

MEASLES

This is a disease of children of age 2-8 years.

I. Transmission by droplets through the respiratory route. Catarrhal symptoms, are followed by the appearance of maculopapular rash on the 4th day. Starting from the face and **behind ears**, then spreading to the trunk and limbs.

The macules coalesce to form large irregular lesion with characteristic morbilliform pattern and they fade in the 6th to 10th day to leave brownish stains and desquamation. Hemorrhagic to vesicular to bullous lesions can also develop.

Diagnosis is by characteristic exanthem with fever catarrhal symptoms and presence of bluish white spots with bright red areola opposite the premolar tooth on the buccal mucosa **(KOPLIK SPOTS).** Also by specific measures antibodies/ by isolation.

Treatment and Prevention: Bed rest with symptomatic management. Vaccination is now advisable at 9 months of age.

Complications: Bronchopneumonia, enteritis, otitis media and most seriously, SSPE (subacute sclerosing pan encephalitis).

RUBELLA

It is an RNA virus belonging either to the group of togavirus family or to the paramyxoviruses.

I. *Transmission*—By droplet infection.

II. A pale pink morbiliform eruption appears without any prodrome, over the face and very rapidly (same day) spreads over to the trunk and limbs and disappears over the neck in 3-4 days. Dull red macules or petechiae are present in the oral mucosa **(Forschheimier sign)** but no koplik spots.

Congenital Rubella form an infection during the 1st trimester of pregnancy can cause: **Rubella Triad (cataract, deafness and cardiac malformations)** with glaucoma, mental retardation, microcephaly, jaundice and purpura with hyperpigmentation of forehead, cheeks and umbilicus. Chronic urticaria/reticulate erythema may be present.

Diagnosis by serology of blood at onset of rash and 7-10 days later to show positive hemagglutination. IgM antibodies specific to rubella in neonates is positive

Treatment—Not specific. Only symptomatic management suffices.

MULTIPLE CHOICE QUESTIONS

1. **A patient made a self-diagnosis of athlete's foot (tinea pedis) and began using a product advertised on television. The condition improved but did not clear and then the patient showed himself a Dermatologist. A skin scraping was sent to the laboratory for culture, including culture for fungi. The fungal culture yielded a slow growing colony, which produced a few small micro-conidia. This is consistent with isolation of dermatophyte of the genera:**
   - A. Trichophyton
   - B. Microsporum
   - C. Epidermophyton
   - D. Trichosporon
2. **A 24-year-old man had multiple, small hypopigmented macules on the upper chest and back for the last three months. The macules were circular, arranged around follicles and many had coalesced to form large sheets. The surface of the macules showed fine scaling. He had similar lesions one year ago, which subsided with treatment. The most appropriate investigation to confirm the diagnosis is:**
   - A. Potassium hydroxide preparation of scales
   - B. Slit skin smear from dicrete macules
   - C. Tzanck test
   - D. Skin biopsy of coalesced macules
3. **A 22-year-old male patient presents with a complaint of severe itching and white scaly lesions in the groin for past one month. Which of the following is most likely to be the causative agent?**
   - A. Trichophyton rubrum
   - B. Candida albicans
   - C. Candida glabrata
   - D. Malassezia furfur
4. **A patient, resident of Himachal Pradesh presented with a series of ulcers in a row, on his right leg. The biopsy from the affected area was taken and cultured on Sabauraud's Dextrose agar. What would be the most likely causative organism?**
   - A. Sporothrix schenckii
   - B. Cladoporium spp.
   - C. Pseudoallescheria boydii
   - D. Nocardia brasiliensis
5. **An elderly diabetic has left sided orbital cellulites, CT scan of paranasal sinuses shows evidence of left maxillary sinusitis. Gram stained smear of the orbital exudates shows irregularly branching sepate hyphae. The following is the most likely aetiological agent:**
   - A. Aspergillus
   - B. Rhizopus
   - C. Mucor
   - D. Candida
6. **'Circle of Hebra' is seen in:**
   - A. Candidasis
   - B. Mucormycosis
   - C. Scabies
   - D. SLE

1 A 2 A 3 A 4 A 5 C 6 C

7. Organisms causing eumycetoma–all *except*:
A. Pseudoallescheria boydii
B. Nocardia brasiliensis
C. Madurella mycetomatis
D. Exophiala mycetomatis

8. All are true of lupus vulgaris *except*:
A. Apple jelly nodules are seen on diascopy
B. Squamous cell carcinoma can develop in long standing cases
C. Lesions show atrophy at one end
D. Montoux test is usually negative

9. Buruli's ulcer is due to infection with:
A. Mycobacterium balneio
B. Mycobacterium ulcerans
C. Mycobacterium kansasi
D. M. avium complex

10. Interval between primary infection and lesions of tertiary syphilis is:
A. 4-6 weeks
B. 6 months
C. 3 years
D. 7 years

11. Pityrosporum orbiculare (causing Tinia versicolor) causes hypopigmentation of skin due to:
A. Direct damage to melanocytes
B. Utilization of substrate DOPA by the yeast
C. Production of azelaic acid which inhibits melanocyte tyrosinase
D. Inhibition of melamosome transfer

12. Erythrasma is caused by:
A. Corynebacterium minutissimum
B. C. diphtheriae
C. C. ulcerans
D. C. vaginale

13. SSS syndrome is due to phage type:
A. 71 B. 80
C. 90 D. 104

14. "Creeping eruption" is caused due to larvae of:
A. Ankylostoma caninum
B. Strongyloidis stercoralis
C. Guinea worm
D. Enterobius vernicularis

15. All of the following can be used to treat post kala azar leishmaniasis *except*:
A. Antimonials
B. Rifampicin
C. Ketoconazole
D. Chloroquine

16. The average number of adult female mites in an adult patient of scabies is:
A. 1-2 B. 5-10
C. 10-14 D. 100-200

17. Treatment of choice for scabies in a 3-month-old infant boy is:
A. 25% benzyl benzoate lotion
B. 1% GBHC lotion
C. 5% topical; permetherin cream
D. Oral ivermectin 200 μg/kg single dose

18. Apple jelly nodules appearance on diascopy is seen in:
A. Psoriasis vulgaris
B. Pemphigus vulgaris
C. Lupus vulgaris
D. Verruca vulgaris

19. "Black dot" effect is seen in:
A. Alopecia areata
B. Pediculosis capitis
C. Tinea capitis due to T. tonsurans
D. Tinea capitis due to T. violaceum

7 B 8 D 9 B 10 D 11 C 12 A 13 A 14 A 15 D 16 C 17 C
18 C 19 C

20. **Favus is a characteristic variety of tinea capitis seen in:**
A. Andhra Pradesh
B. Assam
C. Kerala
D. Kashmir

21. **Papulovesicular eruptions on face trunk, palms and soles in a 9-month-old infant are most likely due to:**
A. Atopic dermatitis
B. Measles
C. Drug reaction
D. Seborrhoeic dermatitis
E. Scabies

22. **Drug of choice for cutaneuos sporotrichosis is:**
A. Amphotericin B
B. Saturated solution of potassium iodide
C. Grieseofulvin
D. Miconazole

23. **Treatment of choice for Norwegian scabies is:**
A. GBHC 1%
B. Permethrin 5%
C. Ivermectin
D. Penicillin

24. **Virchow cells are found in:**
A. Syphilis
B. Lichen planus
C. Leprosy
D. Cutaneous leishmaniasis

25. **Tinea capitis caused by all of the following fluoresces under Wood's light *except*:**
A. T. schoenleinii
B. M. canis
C. M. audouinii
D. T. tonsurans

26. **All of the following are true of Majocchi's granuloma *except*:**
A. It is a type of dermatophyte infection
B. Patients usually presents with one or more tender boggy papules on plagues on the legs
C. Treatment consists of oral antifungal agents
D. Trichoplayton rubrum or T. mentageophytes are the species most commonly isolated from these lesions
E. Oral corticosteorids are the drug of choice

27. **Diseases transmitted by body louse all *except*:**
A. Trench fever
B. Q. fever
C. Relapsing fever
D. Epidemic typhus

28. **Ramsay Hunt syndrome is zoster of:**
A. Ciliary ganglion
B. Otic ganglion
C. Submandibular ganglion
D. Geniculate ganglion

29. **The optimum duration treatment with systemic antifungal drugs in a case of tinea unguum of the finger of nails is:**
A. 15 days
B. 1 month
C. 3 months
D. 6 months

30. **Adamson's fringe is due to .... infection:**
A. Bacterial
B. Viral
C. Fungal
D. Protozoal

31. **Regarding athlete's foot which is:**
A. 4th toe web commonly involved
B. Severe itching
C. Caused by trichophyton mentagrophyte
D. Hyperhydrosis is present
E. All of the above

20 D 21 E 22 B 23 C 24 C 25 D 26 E 27 B 28 D 29 C 30 C 31 E

32. Framboesia of pain is caused by:
A. Leishmania tropica
B. Treponema pertunae
C. Toxocora canis
D. Tinea capitis

33. Bockhart's impetigo is characterized by following *except*:
A. Lesions on legs, thighs and forearms
B. Staphylococcal infection
C. Scarring and falling of hair
D. Treatment of impetigo contagiosa

34. In Ridley Jopling classification of leprosy which of the following term is not used:
A. Lepromatous leprosy
B. Borderline leprosy
C. Indeterminate leprosy
D. Histoid leprosy

35. A 10-year-old child complaining of pustular lesions for 1 year duration shows dark crusted lesions superficial scars on legs. The most likely diagnosis is:
A. Impetigo contagiosa
B. Bockhart's impetigo
C. Tropical sores
D. Ecthyma

36. Which of the following HSV type is associated with Kaposi's sarcoma?
A. HSV–3
B. HSV–5
C. HSV–7
D. HSV–8

37. Treatment of choice for persistent palmo-plantar pustulosis:
A. Methotrexate
B. PUVA
C. Oral retinoids
D. Ingrams regimen

38. All of the following are used to treat pediculosis of eyelashes *except*:
A. Yellow oxide of mercury
B. Petrolatum
C. Physostigmine ointment
D. 1% permethrin

39. Treatment of choice for single lesion of leprosy (WHO):
A. ROM therapy
B. 6 months of PB–MDT
C. Immunotherapy
D. No treatment required®just observe

40. Inverted saucer appearance in leprosy is seen in:
A. Borderline leprosy
B. Tuberculoid leprosy
C. Lepromatous leprosy
D. Borderline tuberculoid leprosy

41. Regimen of choice for cutaneous tuberculosis in HIV is (WHO):
A. 2 months intensive + 7 months maintenance
B. 2 months + 4 months
C. 2 months + 6 months

42. Most common cause of "FAVUS" is:
A. Trichophyton rubrum
B. Trichophyton schoenleinii
C. Microsporun canis
D. Epidermophyton floccosum

43. Most common cause of athletes foot:
A. Histoplasma capsulatum
B. Pityrosporum ovale
C. Corynebacterium minutiimum
D. Trichophyton rubrum

---

32 B 33 C 34 C,D 35 C 36 D 37 A,C 38 D 39 A 40 A 41 A 42 B
43 D

44. P. versicolor is caused by:
A. M. furfur
B. T. rubrum
C. C. albicans
D. Cryptococcus neoformans

45. Tinea capitis is caused by all *except*:
A. Epidermophyton floccosum
B. Trichophyton tonsurans
C. Microsporon audoninii
D. Trichophyton violaceum

46. Endothrix type of Tinea capitis is caused by all *except*:
A. Trichophyton tonsurans
B. Trichophyton violaceum
C. Tricho soudanense
D. Trichophyton schoenleinii

47. Kerion is a:
A. Type of bacterial folliculitis
B. Inflammatory fungal infection of scalp
C. Endothrix type of Tinea capitis
D. Inflammatory type of tinea capitis

48. White peidra is caused by:
A. Peidraia hortae
B. Trichosporon beigelii
C. Trichophyton violaceun
D. Microsporon canis

49. Dimorphic fungi cause all of the following *except*:
A. Sporotrichosis
B. Histoplasmosis
C. Paracoccidioimycosis
D. Blastomycosis
E. Candidiasis

50. Mucormycosis occurs in:
A. Diabetic ketoacidosis
B. Ureamia
C. Corticosteroid therapy
D. Malnutrition
E. All of the above

51. Moth eaten alopecia is characteristic of:
A. Tinea capitis
B. Secondary syphilis
C. Lupus vulgaris
D. Telogen effeuvium

52. Corynebacterium minutissimum causes:
A. Acne rosacea
B. Erysipelas
C. Erythrasma
D. Erysipeloid

53. Erisepalas is caused by:
A. B-haemolytic streptococcus
B. Erysipelothrix rhusiopapathae
C. Staph aureus
D. Corynebacterium minutissimum

54. Strength of benzyl benzoate used to treat scabies:
A. 10%
B. 15%
C. 20%
D. 25%

55. Strength of gama-benzene hexachloride used to treat scabies:
A. 1% B. 2%
C. 5% D. 10%

56. Disease transmitted by body louse:
A. Trench fever
B. Q. fever
C. Relapsing fever
D. Epidemic typhus

57. Most suitable site for demonstration of the mite in scabies is:
A. Papule
B. Superficial ulcer
C. Ends of burrow
D. Papulo pustule

---

44 A 45 A 46 B 47 B 48 B 49 E 50 E 51 B 52 C 53 A 54 D
55 A 56 B 57 C

58. Sycosis barbae is caused by:
A. Staphylococcus aureus
B. Streptococcus pyogenes
C. Trichophyton rubrum
D. Microsporum canis

59. All are types of cutaneous tuberculosis *except*:
A. Lupus vulgaris
B. Scrofuloderma
C. Tuberculosis verrucosa cutis
D. Lupus pernio

60. Swimming pool granuloma results from:
A. Chlamydia trachomatis
B. Mycobacterium tuberculosis
C. Mycobacteruim marinum
D. Guinea worm

61. Following region is most frequently affected by herpes zoster:
A. Cervical
B. Dorso lumbar
C. Thoracic
D. Sacral

62. Herpangina is caused by:
A. Herpes simplex virus
B. Coxsackie A
C. Ebstein bar virus
D. Varicella zoster virus

63. All result from viral infection *except*:
A. Filiform warts
B. Mosaic plantar warts
C. Butchers wart
D. Plane warts

64. Forchheimers spots are seen in:
A. Measles
B. Rubella
C. Varicella
D. ECHO virus infections

65. Treatment of choice for primary herpes simplex is:
A. Acyclovir
B. Photo inactivation
C. Thalidomide
D. Silver sulphadizine

66. All of the following organs are involved in leprosy *except*:
A. Liver B. Testes
C. Bones D. Brain
E. Eyes

67. Histoid leprosy is a type of:
A. Lepromatous leprosy
B. Borderline leprosy
C. Tuberculoid leprosy
D. Neither of the above

68. Following are true of lepromatous leprosy *except*:
A. Multiple symmetrical lesions
B. Leonine facies
C. Madarosis
D. Positive lepromin test

69. The following quinolones are effective in leprosy *except*:
A. Pefloxacin B. Sparfloxacin
C. Ciprofloxacin D. Sparfloxacin

70. Corneal ulcer in leprosy is most often due to involvement of:
A. Facial nerve
B. Trigeminal
C. Optic nerve
D. Ophthalmic nerve

71. Globi in slit smear are seen in:
A. Lepromatous leprosy
B. Histoid leprosy
C. Indeterminate leprosy
D. Borderline leprosy

58 C 59 D 60 C 61 C 62 B 63 C 64 B 65 A 66 D 67 A 68 D
69 C 70 A 71 A

72. Which of the following HLA type is associated with tuberculoid hansens?
A. HLA-DR3 B. HLA-DR2
C. HLA-DR4 D. HLA-DW

73. Acid fastness of lepra bacilli is lost but gram positivity is preserved with:
A. Hyaluronic acid
B. Pyridine
C. Pyrimidine
D. Palmitic acid

74. G. Armauer Hansen was a:
A. Microbiologist
B. Pathologist
C. Leprologist
D. Biochemist

75. Hypopigmentation in lesions of leprosy is because of:
A. Competition of lepra bacilli with melanocytes over dopa substrate
B. Damage to melanocytes
C. Anti leprosy drugs
D. Langerhan cell damage

76. The major circulating metabolite of DDS in man is:
A. Mono acetyle dapsone
B. Glucosulfone
C. Di-actyl-dapsone
D. Tri-acetyl-dapsone

77. "Lucio phenomenon" is a type of:
A. Lepromatous leprosy
B. Lepra reaction
C. Borderline leprosy
D. Drug reaction seen in leprosy

78. All of the following is true about Lucio Leprosy *except*:
A. First described in Mexico
B. Diffuse non nodular type of leprosy
C. Skin lesions similar to LL Hansens
D. Thickening of upper eyelids gives patients a sleepy or melancholy look

79. All of the following are true of association of pregnancy with leprosy *except*:
A. Women with incubating leprosy are likely to show overt signs of the disease in pregnancy
B. Nerve function of leprosy patients improves during pregnancy
C. In borderline leprosy upgrading reaction is most likely to occur during puerperium
D. Type 2 reaction (ENL) is most likely to occur in the third trimester and puerperium

80. All are true of thalidomide *except*:
A. Drug of choice for type 2 reaction (ENL)
B. Drug of choice for type 1 reaction
C. It is of no value in type 1 reaction
D. It is teratogenic

8 . All are indications of systemic steroid therapy in leprosy *except*:
A. Neuritis in type 1 reaction
B. Iritis/iridocyclitis
C. Epididymo orchitis
D. Necrotic –ENL reaction
E. Histoid leprosy

82. All are side-effects of clofazimine *except*:
A. Red brown pigmentation of skin and conjunctival
B. Red colouration of urine, stools, sputum, sweat and tears
C. Dryness of skin
D. Gastrointestinal disturbance
E. Steven Johnson syndrome

72 A 73 B 74 B 75 A 76 A 77 B 78 C 79 B 80 B 81 E 82 E

83. Flu like syndrome is a side-effect of:
A. Daily rifampicin therapy
B. Intermittent rifampicin therapy
C. Dapsone
D. Clofazimine

84. Methaemoglobinaemia is a side-effect:
A. Dapsone
B. Daily rifampicin therapy
C. Intermittent rifampicin therapy
D. Thalidomide

85. All are true of ENL reaction *except*:
A. It is a type of type III hypersensitivity reaction
B. Occurs in lepromatous leprosy
C. Characterised by crops of erythematous evanescent tender nodules
D. Systemic disturbance is usual
E. Occurs usually during first 6 months of therapy

86. All are newer drugs recommended for treatment of leprosy *except*:
A. Sparfloxacin
B. Minocycline
C. Ofloxacin
D. Dapsone
E. Moxifloxacin

87. The morphological index (MI) of a leprosy patient is calculated after examination red staining elements lying singly in a slit-skin smear:
A. 100 B. 200
C. 300 D. 50

88. The MI (morphological index) of a lepromatous patient is between:
A. 25-50
B. 50-75
C. 25-75
D. 75-100

89. All are high endemic areas for leprosy in India *except*:
A. West Bengal
B. Eastern Uttar Pradesh
C. Rajasthan
D. Bihar
E. Tamilnadu

90. Low endemic areas are described as those having incidence of leprosy:
A. <1-5/1000 B. <1/1000
C. <5/1000 D. <10/1000

91. All of the following are types of secondary syphilis rash in adults *except*:
A. Maculo papular
B. Follicular
C. Corymbose
D. Vesiculo bullous
E. Pustular

92. Treatment of choice of pediculosis corporis is:
A. 1% permethium application
B. Benzyl benzoate application
C. 5% permethium application
D. Laundering and ironing of clothes

93. Most common form of actinomycosis:
A. Cervico facial
B. Thoracic
C. Axillary
D. Abdominal

94. Virchow cells are:
A. Histiocytes B. Melanocytes
C. Langerhan cells D. Keratinocytes

95. The following systemic drugs can be used for the treatment of warts:
A. Doxycycline
B. Colchicine
C. Griseofulvin
D. None of the above

83 B 84 A 85 E 86 D 87 B 88 C 89 C 90 B 91 D 92 D 93 A
94 A 95 C

96. Antibiotic effect of griseofulvin on dermatophytes is apparently on:

A. Mature cells
B. Actively metabolising cells
C. Spores
D. Microconidia

97. The optimum duration of treatment of tinea unguium with griseofulvin is:

A. 15 days
B. 1 month
C. 3 months
D. 6 months

98. Best treatment of scabies in an infant is:

A. 25% benzyl benzoate
B. 1% gamma aninobenzoic
C. Crotamiton
D. Sulphur

99. Average duration of treatment in multibacillary leprosy is:

A. 2 years
B. 1 year
C. 5 years
D. Life long

100. Dose of acyclovir in a patient suffering from herpes zoster is:

A. 200 mg, five times a day for 2 days
B. 400 mg, five times a day for 3 days
C. 800 mg, five times a day for 5 days
D. 600 mg, five times a day for 5 days

101. Treatment of choice for Bushke Lowenstein syndrome is:

A. Cryosurgery
B. Keratolytics
C. U-V rays
D. Dapsone

102. Milker's nodule:

A. Is pre-malignant
B. Is usually painful
C. Is characterized by eosinophilic cytoplasmic inclusion bodies
D. None of the above

103. A person is suffering from lepromatosis leprosy—what will you advise his family members?

A. Full course of MD-MDT
B. Only daily rifampicin
C. To isolate the patient
D. Chemoprophylaxis is not required

104. All true regarding leprosy and pregnancy *except*:

A. Nerve function deteriorates during pregnancy
B. Type 2 reaction (ENL) is most likely to occur in the third trimester and puerperium
C. MDT should be discontinued
D. Upgrading reaction is likely to occur during puerperium in borderline leprosy

105. Follow-up after completion of MDT is advised:

A. In all multibacillary patients
B. Only in those with initial bacteriological index > 4 +
C. For 1 year in paucibacillary and 5 years in multibacillary patients
D. There is no need for follow-up

106. Lazarine leprosy:

A. Is a type of lepromatous leprosy
B. Seen in immunocompromised individuals
C. Seen only in Mexico
D. Systemic corticosteroids are a must for treatment

96 B 97 D 98 D 99 B 100 C 101 A 102 C 103 D 104 C 105 D 106 A

107. All true of morphological index in leprosy *except*:
- **A.** It is calculated after examining 100 red staining elements lying singly in a skin slit smear
- **B.** The MI of a lepromatous patient is between 25-75
- **C.** It is useful in assessing response to treatment
- **D.** In lepromatous leprosy, it should reach zero in 4-6 weeks on multi-drug therapy.

108. Bachman test is a skin for:
- **A.** Histoplasmosis
- **B.** Trichinosis
- **C.** Cysticercosis
- **D.** Sarcoidosis

109. The correct concentration of potassium hydroxide for demonstrating the dermatophyte is:
- **A.** 0.5% **B.** 2%
- **C.** 5% **D.** 10%

110. The optimum time required for culturing dermatophytes is:
- **A.** 24 weeks **B.** 48 hours
- **C.** 1 week **D.** 2 weeks

111. Mupirocin (previously called pseudomonic acid) acid as topical anti-infective competes with amino acid .... for enzyme binding sites:
- **A.** Glycine
- **B.** Lysine
- **C.** Isoleucine
- **D.** Phenylalanine

112. Spaghetti and meatballs or hot dogs and baked beans are seen in:
- **A.** Pemphigus
- **B.** Scalded skin syndrome
- **C.** Tinea versicolor
- **D.** Lichen planus

113. Uses of woods light includes:
- **A.** Urine examination in poryphyria
- **B.** Examination of hair in T. capitis
- **C.** Sclerema
- **D.** Tinea cruris

114. Which of the following is true of molluscum contagiosum?
- **A.** Treatment is expiration
- **B.** Can be transmitted sexually
- **C.** Central umbilication
- **D.** All of the above

115. Treatment of tinea veriscolor:
- **A.** Clotrimazole
- **B.** Sodium sulphite
- **C.** Selenium sulphide
- **D.** Miconazole
- **E.** All of the above

116. In a dermatophytosis the duration of griseofulvin therapy is about:
- **A.** Two months
- **B.** One month
- **C.** Depends on the blood levels of drug achieved
- **D.** Depends on the renewal time of the stratum corneum involved

117. A 2-year-old child with an upper respiratory infection suddenly develops a bluish red ill-defined warm oedematous plaque on face. This picture is typical of:
- **A.** Erysipelas
- **B.** Anthrax
- **C.** Disseminated intravascular coagulation
- **D.** Haemophilus influenzae cellulitis

107 B 108 B 109 D 110 D 111 C 112 C 113 B 114 D 115 E 116 D 117 D

118. Verruca vulgaris:
A. Autoinoculable
B. Contagious
C. Spontaneously disappear
D. All of the above

119. Erythrasma would most likely be found in the:
A. Face
B. Toewebs
C. Trunk
D. Elbows

120. Most common site for erysipelas:
A. Trunk
B. Legs
C. Arms
D. Face and head

121. Pitted keratolysis is caused by:
A. Bacteria
B. Viruses
C. Fungus
D. Rickettsia

122. Deep fungal infection is caused by all *except*:
A. Cryptococcus
B. Streptothrix
C. Histoplasma
D. Nocardia

123. Causative organisms of maduramycetoma is:
A. Nocardia brasiliense
B. Aspergillus flavus
C. Histoplasma flavus
D. H. dubosii

124. Which of the following is not true about herpangina?
A. Exhibits pharyngeal vesicles and ulcers
B. Tends to occur in the winter
C. Is caused by coxsackie virus
D. Is usually a mild febrile illness

125. The rash in measles occurs first in the .... region.
A. Forehead
B. Post auricular
C. Chest
D. Neck

126. Griseofulvin is not useful in one of the following:
A. Tinea capitis
B. Tinea cruris
C. Tinea versicolor
D. Tinea pedis

127. Hidradenitis suppurativa is most often due to:
A. Str. pyogenes
B. Staph. aureus
C. Treponema pallidum
D. Candida ablicans

128. The following drugs are effective in treatment of mycetoma *except*:
A. Erythromycin
B. Tetracycline
C. Sulfonamides
D. Dapsone

129. Dhobi's itch is:
A. Tinea corporis
B. Tinea cruris
C. Tinea barbae
D. Tinea capitis

130. Copra itch is caused by:
A. Soft tick
B. Hard tick
C. Flea
D. Mite

131. Bed bug is also known as:
A. Cimex lectularis
B. Ixodes
C. Tryoglyhus langior
D. Trombicula irritans

118 D 119 B 120 D 121 A 122 B 123 A 124 B 125 B 126 C 127 B 128 A 129 B 130 D 131 A

132. Demodex folliculorum produces itching lesions on:

A. Trunk
B. Face
C. Palm creases
D. Sole creases

133. Delhi boil is caused by:

A. Staph. aureus
B. Str. pyogenes
C. Leishmania tropica
D. Candida albicans

134. Post herpetic neuralgia commonly develop in patients of the following age group:

A. Infants
B. School going children
C. 20-30 years
D. Above 40 years

135. Features of rash in herpes zoster include each of the following *except*:

A. Follows a nerve distribution
B. May involve one or more dermatomes
C. Always appears in patches where the cutaneous nerves branch to the skin
D. On the thorax and abdomen, the linear vesicular rash stops sharply at the midline

136. Erythema infectiosum is caused by:

A. Echoviruses
B. Paroviruses
C. Paramyxovirus
D. Coxsackie virus

137. "Slapped cheek" appearance is typically seen in:

A. Mumps
B. Rubella
C. Erythema infectiosum
D. Exanthema sabitum

138. Erythema chronicum migrans is caused by:

A. Spirochaetes
B. Internal malignancy
C. Zinc deficiency
D. Rheumatic fever

139. Most common cause of angular chelitis is:

A. Candidiasis
B. Mechanical
C. Syphilis
D. Vitamin deficiency

132 B 133 C 134 D 135 C 136 B 137 C 138 A 139 A

Chapter 3

Papulosquamous Disorders

- Psoriasis.
- Lichen planus.
- Pityriasis rosea.
- Pityriasis rubra pilaris.
- Pityriasis lichenoides.
- Parapsoriasis.
- Seborrhoeic dermatitis.
- Nummular dermatitis.
- Drug eruptions.

Psoriasis

It is a common, genetically determined, inflammatory skin disorder of unknown cause, usually characterized by well defined, raised, erythematous, scaly plaques, preferentially localized to the extensors. It affects approximately **2%** of the general population. A positive **family history is present in 40%** of the patients. A bimodal pattern of onset has been reported with the peak ages of onset being between 16-22 years and 57-60 years.

Natural History

Psoriasis is a chronic disorder with unpredictable remissions and relapses. Single episodes are distinctly uncommon. The disease has a considerable psychological impact on the affected individual.

Etiopathogenesis

The exact etiology of psoriasis is uncertain and appears to be multifactorial. Role of genetic factors is thought to be important, though no single gene has been clearly implicated. Other factors like autoimmunity, superantigens, physical, chemical or UV injury have been thought to be responsible for the hyperproliferative state evident in psoriatic plaques.

Two Types of Psoriasis—Type 1 and 2.

Strongest genetic link is—**HLA Cw6.**

Genetic loci –**Psor 1 to 6**.

Strongest link with Psor 1 **(chromosome 6).**

- A child with one affected parent has 15% chance of developing the disease, but if both the parents are affected, then the risk increases to 50%. With one sibling—24%. Both parents with one sibling—83%.
- Early onset—type I is associated with HLA-Cw-6.
- Late onset—type II is associated with HLA-Cw-2.

Drugs: Various drugs are associated with psoriasis:

- Lithium.
- Beta-blockers.
- Anti-malarials.
- Withdrawal of systemically administered corticosteroids.
- Clonidine.
- Trazodone.
- Amidarone.
- ACE inhibitors.

- Gemfibrozil.
- Terfinadine.
- NSAIDS.

HYPER PROLIFERATION OF KERATINOCYTES

- The finding of greatly enhanced keratinocytes proliferation in psoriasis is at least in part due to a reduced cell cycle time **(311 hours to 36 hours).**
- The abnormality in psoriatic epidermis appears to be the result of an increased recruitment of cycling cells from the resting fraction, thus producing an increased growth fraction. The growth fraction normal—60% approaches 100%.

INFLAMMATION/ROLE OF T CELLS

Psoriasis is now thought of an immunological disease driven by activated memory T cells. There are two populations of T cells:

- **Dermal T cells,** which are primarily, **CD-4 Cells.**
- **Epidermal T cells** which are primarily **CD-8 Cells.**

ROLE OF SUPER ANTIGENS

- Super antigens are highly potent stimulators of T cells, monocytes and macrophages, binding with T cells do not require APC.
- Globular proteins of 22-29 Dalton, very resistant to destruction.
- Easily absorbable by epithelium as immunologically in tact protein.

Morphological Variants

1. *Chronic plaque psoriasis* is characterized by well demarcated, salmon pink coloured, papules and plaques, covered with silvery white scales which on removal, show minute bleeding points **(Auspitz sign and Grattage test).** The plaques are symmetrically distributed on the extensor aspects, especially the elbows and the knees. New lesions occur at the site of trauma (Koebner's phenomenon).
2. *Guttate (exanthemic psoriasis):* This form is commonly seen in infants and children. Multiple 'rain drop' lesions suddenly appear on the trunk and the limbs and are usually preceded by a streptococcal sore throat.
3. *Inverse psoriasis:* It is characterized by well demarcated, erythematous lesions symmetrically distributed over the flexural areas, including the axillae, groins, perineum and perianal areas. They are often confused with intertrigo, candidiasis and dermatophytic infection (also known as **white psoriasis**).
4. *Erythrodermic psoriasis:* In this, the disease involves more than 90% of the body surface area with widespread scaling and erythema. Chronic lesions may evolve gradually into an extensive disease. The second form may be a part of the spectrum of unstable psoriasis implying a loss of control over the disease.
5. *Palmoplantar psoriasis:* There are localized, erythematous, scaly plaques over the palms and soles, preferentially involving the thenar and hypothenar eminences with no other evidence of proriasis elsewhere.
6. *Scalp psoriasis:* Multiple, discrete plaques involving gradually entire scalp can occur. **Pityriasis amiantacea** characterized by masses of adherent silvery scales with occasional loss of hair may be seen.
7. *Nail psoriasis* is characterized by fine pitting, distal onycholysis, subungual hyperkeratosis, oil drop sign or salmon patch.
8. *Psoriatic arthropathy:* It is a mono or an asymmetric oligoarthritis usually involving the joints of upper limb. Distal interphalangeal or sacroiliac joints are also involved. Arthritis mutilans is a severe destructive form of the disease.

9. *Sebopsoriasis:* It is a variant which shows features of both psoriasis and seborhoeic dermatitis. It is speculated that lipophilic yeasts may play a pathogenic role.
10. *Pustular psoriasis:* It is characterized by the appearance of macroscopic pustules. It may be of two types. In the localised form, it is confined to hands and feet and tends to be chronic. In the generalized form, the whole body may be involved and the course is subacute, acute or even fulminating and life threatening.

Nail

The characteristic nail changes/abnormal nail findings seen in psoriasis: Are found in 25-50% of psoriatics. These changes include nail pitting, discoloration, onycholysis, subungual hyperkeratosis, and nail deformity.

- Nail changes in psoriasis ranges from minor defects in the nail plate (pits) to severe alterations of the nail organ (onychodystrophy) and loss of the nail plate when the pustular forms of psoriasis involve the nail.
- Due to defective keratinization of the dorsal side of the proximal nail fold, pits are evident within the nail plate.
- Yellowish macules beneath the nail plate caused by psoriatic processes located in the nail bed (Oil drop sign).
- The nail matrix involvement leads to severe onychodystrophy.
- In pustular psoriasis, the nail changes consist of subungual pustules of the nail bed or the nail matrix.
- In pustular psoriasis of the palms and soles, nail changes are rare.
- Nail changes are more frequent in patients with arthritis.

Psoriatic Arthritis

An estimated 5-10% of patients with psoriasis suffer from psoriatic arthritis. The arthritis may precede, accompany, or, more commonly, follow the skin disease.

There are five types of psoriatic arthritis:

- Asymmetric (60-70%).
- Symmetric polyarthritis (15%).
- Distal interphalangeal joint (DIP) disease (5%).
- Destructive arthritis (5%) *(arthritis mutilans, "opera glass" deformity.*
- Axial arthritis (5%).

Clinically, asymmetric arthritis, the most common type, usually involves one or several joints of the fingers or toes. The appearance of this type of arthritis can be similar to subacute gout and include *"sausage-like"* swelling of a digit due to involvement of the proximal and DIP joints and flexor sheath.

Symmetric polyarthritis resembles rheumatoid arthritis, but tests for rheumatoid factor are negative and and the condition is clinically less severe than rheumatoid-arthritis. Although not common, DIP joint disease of hands and feet is the most characteristic presentation of arthritis with psoriasis. Destructive arthritis *(arthritis mutilans)* is a severely deforming arthritis involving predominantly fingers and toes. Gross osteolysis of the small bones of the hands and feet can result in shortening, subluxations, and, in' severe cases, telescoping of the digits, resulting in an *"opera glass" deformity.*

Several factors are implicated in provoking or exacerbating psoriasis. New lesions may occur at the site of trauma (Koebner phenomenon). Various infections, most importantly, streptococcal infection may play a role. Sunlight, though generally beneficial, may occasionally exacerbate the disease. Hypocalcemia, stress, smoking and alcohol also exacerbate the disease. Various drugs including lithium, beta-blockers, antimalarials amiodarone also aggravate or precipitate psoriasis.

Treatment

A large number of treatment options are available with topical modalities being used for mild psoriasis and systemic options for moderate to severe disease. Emollients or keratolytics are useful forms of treatment. Tar preparations and dithranol have been in use for many years for chronic plaque psoriasis. They are effective because of their antimitotic action. Topical corticosteroids are very useful for psoriasis on delicate areas like face, flexures and genitalia. They are effective, but continued use is related to tachyphylaxis, systemic side effects and rebound flare. Topical vitamin D3 analogues especially calcipotriol ointment have an efficacy equivalent to topical steroids with fewer side effects.

Ultraviolet light in the form of psoralen + UVA therapy (PUVA) has been used for a large number of patients. UVB therapy alone or with tar baths is also an effective mode of therapy. For arthropathy and widespread disease such as erythroderma systemic immunosuppressive and cytotoxic therapies like methotrexate, cyclosporin etc. or agents like retinoids found to be useful under close specialist care.

1. **Localised disease**—20 to 30% area–**Topical** therapy.
   Goeckerman regimen–Tar + UVB.
   Ingram regimen–Anthralin.
   Newer topical–Calcipotriol,tacrolimus, tazarotene.
2. **Generalised**
   Systemic–PUVA, Nb UVB.
   Methotrexate (pulse regimen once a week **Weinstein—Frost regimen)**, Cyclosporine.
   Biological therapy:
   DOC
   Guttate—Antibiotics.
   Pustular—Retinoids, methotrexate.
   Erythrodermic—Methotrexate.

Treatment

Large number of treatment options are available for the treatment of psoriasis, with topical modalities being used for mild psoriasis and systemic options for moderate to severe disease.

Topical Treatment

Anthralin:

A. **Classical anthralin therapy:** Starts using low concentrations (0.05 to 0.1%) incorporated in petrolatum or zinc paste and given once daily.

B. **Short-contact treatment:** Higher concentrations of anthralin (1 to 5%) in water-soluble vehicles are applied to the lesions for a short period of time (usually 10 to 20 min).

Vitamin D3 Analogues

Soon after the introduction of calcipotriol (calcipotriene)—the first vitamin D3 analogue-it became a widely used remedy for plaque psoriasis. It has also been shown that the active hormone *1,25-dihydroxyvitamin D3 (calcitriol)* is an effective therapy for psoriasis when used as topical or systemic treatment.

MOA: **NF-kB protein** in lymphocytes, leading to a reduced transcription of IL-2. Inhibit production of IL-6 from cytokine-stimulated human dermal microvascular endothelial.

Tazarotene induces upregulation of tazarotene-induced-gene 1 (TIG1) in skin.

Treatment with Ultraviolet Light

Photochemotherapy (PUVA)

Parrish 1974, cross-linking bifunctional photoadducts 8-methoxypsoralen (8-MOP) or trimethoxypsoralen at a constant dose (0.6 to 0.8 mg/kg) and variable doses of UVA, depending on the sensitivity of the patient. Approximately 2 hours after ingestion of the psoralen, UVA is started, usually at a dose of 1 J/cm2, adjusting upward for skin type. The UVA dose is increased by sub-erythematous amounts, generally ranging from 0.5 to 1.5 J/cm2. The dose of UVA for a given treatment should not lead to brisk erythema.

Treatments are performed two or three times a week, or, under a more intensive protocol, four times a week.

Clearing occurs after **19 to 25** treatments.

Bath PUVA

First described by Fischer and Alsins in 1976, this is another way to deliver the photosensitizer (8-MOP or 5-MOP) to the skin is by addition of these compounds to bath water. Major advantages of bath PUVA are the lack of systemic effects, such as gastrointestinal.

Balneophototherapy

Combination of salt-water bathing and sunlight exposure is an effective treatment for psoriasis. From studies at the Dead Sea, it became clear that highly concentrated salt water (>20%) together with UVB light is most effective. A possible mechanism of concentrated salt-water bathing is the elution of biologically active peptide mediators and enzymes such as human leukocyte elastase from the inflamed skin.

Selective UVB Therapy

Narrow-band UVB (311nm), also known as selective UVB phototherapy (SUP), can be performed as monotherapy or preferably in combination with topical treatments such as glucocorticoids, vitamin D3 analogues, or anthralin. SUP is very effective in guttate psoriasis and also improves lesions of the plaque type.

Systemic Treatment

Methotrexate

Methotrexate (MTX, formerly called amethopterin)

MTX inhibits DNA synthesis (S phase of the cell cycle) by competing as a substrate for dihydrofolate reductase.

Dosage of MTX is between 10 and 25 mg once a week. MTX can also be given orally, intravenous or intramuscularly, using a dosing schedule in which 5 mg is given every 12 hours over a 36-hour period.

Folinic acid rescue (25 mg of leucovorin intramuscularly) should be performed, preferably within the first 4 hours.

Cyclosporine

This is a cyclic polypeptide produced by a fungus. It is an immunosuppressive agent widely used for the prevention of graft rejection. After penetration into the cell by a putative receptor, cyclosporine binds to cyclophilin, a member of the immunophilin group.

Retinoids

Etretinate, a derivative of vitamin A, was the first retinoid compound routinely used for the treatment of psoriasis. Retinoids regulate growth and terminal differentiation of keratinocytes, thereby normalizing the hyperproliferative state in psoriasis. Etretinate has now been replaced by acitretin, an equally effective metabolite of etretinate, in many countries. The half-life of etretinate is about 100 days and that of acitretin 2 to 3 days.

Etretinate and acitretin are clinically effective in pustular forms of psoriasis, including generalized pustular psoriasis and pustulosis palmaris et plantaris.

Fumaric Acid Esters

Liarozole

Liarozole, an imidazole-containing compound, is an inhibitor of retinoic acid 4-hydroxylase activity, which can be found in skin. Inhibition of this enzyme results in increased levels of endogenous all-trans-retinoic acid. First clinical studies reveal good clinical responses in patients with severe psoriasis given a 150-mg b.i.d. dose of liarozole. Adverse events were comparable to those seen under systemic retinoid (etretinate/acitretin) therapy.

Combination Therapy

A combination of different therapeutic principles may help to speed resolution of the lesions, reduce adverse events, and reduce overall doses when systemic compounds are used. Several combination regimes have already been established for clinical use, such as topical glucocorticoids with UVB or PUVA, retinoids with PUVA (Re-PUVA), and vitamin D3 analogues with UVB. The combination of coaltar baths, UVB, and anthralin is known as the **Ingram** method. **Goeckerman** in 1925 introduced the widely used combination of coaltar application followed by suberythemic doses of UV-light. Classical anthralin treatment followed by UVB or bath-PUVA is also a very effective combination regimen. More recent studies indicate that combining cyclosporine with calcipotriol or anthralin augments efficacy and reduces cyclosporine dose. Calcipotriol also improves the response to PUVA.

Rotation Treatment

To minimize risk for the patient with severe psoriasis requiring systemic treatment, rotation therapy should be performed. Changing between different compounds on a patient-oriented basis—with respect to individual risk factors, cumulative dose (for MTX), response and duration of therapy—should be performed in intervals. Recently published guidelines for rotation therapy may be helpful in scheduling long-term systemic treatment.

Phototherapy in Psoriasis (Fig. 3.1)

Ultraviolet light is a highly effective treatment, but is carcinogenic (causing mainly squamous cell carcinoma). Accurate monitoring and recording of doses combined with precise calibration of equipment is essential to minimize this risk and maximize efficacy.

UVB comprises light of wavelength 290-320 nm. Traditionally, fluorescent tubes emitting a broad band of wavelengths have been used, but there is a current trend towards use of narrow band UVB, with fluorescent tubes emitting wavelengths of mainly about 311 nm. Eliminating shorter-wavelength UVB increases the efficacy and reduces the risk of burning. It is unclear

T cell-targeted approaches under evaluation in psoriasis

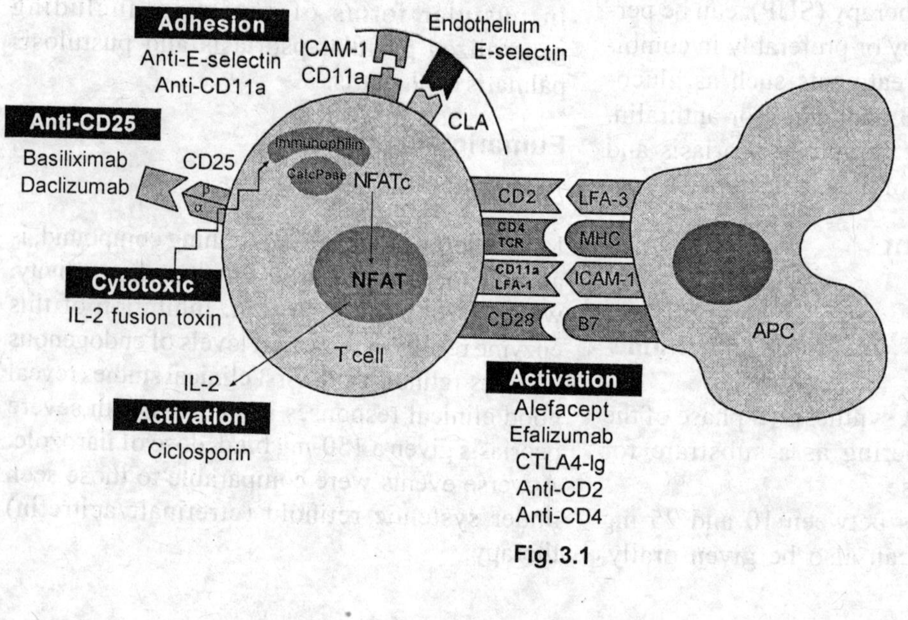

APC—antigen-presenting cell; CalcPase—Calcineurin phosphatase; CLA—Cutaneous lymphocyte-associated antigen; ICAM—Intercellular adhesion molecule; IL—Interleukin; LFA—Lymphocyte function-associated antigen; MHC—Major histocompatibility complex; NFAT—Nuclear factor of activated T cells; TCR—T cell receptor

Source: CEM Griffiths

Fig. 3.1

whether carcinogenesis is reduced compared with treatment with broadband UVB.

UVA (320-400 nm) is minimally effective in the treatment of psoriasis when used alone, but becomes highly effective when combined with photosensitizing psoralen (PUVA). Psoralen is most often administered orally, but can also be applied topically—a useful approach when limited areas such as palms and soles are treated. Bath PUVA involves a 20-minute soak in a bath of psoralen solution before UVA exposure. This avoids systemic exposure to psoralen, and the nausea that some patients experience after oral therapy.

Pityriasis Rosea

It is one of the common acute self-limiting papulosquamous eruption which predominantly affects young adults with minimal constitutional symptoms. Most cases occur between 10-35 years of age and the disease is common during the spring and fall. Etiology is not definitely known. A viral cause, most probably a picornavirus has been implicated. Also, cell mediated immunity, legionella micdadei or the role of drugs has been postulated.

Characteristically, the initial lesion is a solitary, oval, erythematous, scaly **"herald patch",** often seen on the trunk. After 1-2 weeks scaly papules and plaques appear over the trunk, neck and upper arms in a symmetrical **"Christmas tree"** pattern. The eruption usually fades in 4-6 weeks. Various morphological variants like papulovesicular, vesicular, pustular, erythema multiforme like, unilateral, acute purpuric etc. have been reported.

The entity is self limiting and usually no treatment is required. Nevertheless, mild topical steroids and UV exposure may hasten resolution. **(Clinical points—herald patch, Christmas tree pattern, trunk).**

Pityriasis Rubra Pilaris

Pityriasis rubra pilaris (PRP) is a rare disease in which the primary abnormality appears to be hyperproliferation of the epidermis. Five variants have been described. The most common being type I, the classic adult onset.

1. Cephalocaudal fashion.
2. Palms and soles become thickened and yellow, resulting in a well-demarcated, very characteristic "PRP sandal".
3. "Islands of sparing".

PARAPSORIASIS

Parapsoriasis is a term often used to describe slowly evolving, asymptomatic, scaly plaques, often found on the trunk and proximal extremities. Parapsoriasis is divided into small plaque (1-5 cm diameter) and large plaque (5-15 cm diameter) forms. The prognosis of the two types differs, and approximately 10% of cases of large-plaque parapsoriasis eventuate in T-cell lymphoma. Parapsoriasis is resistant to most topical treatments but often responds to phototherapy. It can last months to years. Oral antibiotics (erythromycin or tetracycline) have been suggested, but no controlled studies exist. Phototherapy and even methotrexate have been used for recalcitrant or severe cases.

Pityriasis lichenoides et varioliformis acuta (PLEVA or Mucha-Habermann disease).

Pityriasis lichenoides et varioliformis acuta (PLEVA or Mucha-Habermann disease) is a rare disease characterized by crops of polymorphous lesions on the trunk, thighs, and upper arms. The eruption consists of red-brown papules that can become purpuric, scaly, and even necrotic. The patients usually are asymptomatic, although itching and low-grade fevers and malaise are not uncommon. Individual lesions resolve in several weeks leaving post inflammatory hyper- or hypopigmentation and occasionally scars. The clinical course of PLEVA often waxes and wanes Trt PUVA and doxycycline.

Seborrheic Dermatitis

This is a chronic dermatitis with erythematous sharply marginated lesions, covered with adherent greasy scales and distributed in areas with a rich supply of sebaceous glands i.e. scalp, face and upper trunk. It may affect 1-3 % of general population and is seen in infancy and then in adolescence and adult life. It is rare before puberty and peaks between 18-40 years of age. Males are more commonly affected.

The yeast Malassezia ovale has been implicated as an etiologic factor. The role of sebum in its pathogenesis has not been proved. Seborrhea occurs in association with Parkinsonism, as a marker of HIV infection and in myocardial ischemia, obesity, epilepsy, malabsorption.

Commonly originates in hairy skin and involves **scalp, face, presternal and interscapular area.** The skin in these regions is dull or yellowish red, covered with **greasy scales**. In infants, it may manifest as "cradle cap". **Leiner's** disease is generalized exfoliative dermatitis in an infant secondary to seborrhoeic dermatitis and is associated with C5 deficiency.

In adults, milder form may be seen as dandruff. In the inflammatory form it may extend onto the non-hairy areas and face. Blepharitis and conjunctivitis may also be associated. On the trunk, it may present most commonly as petaloid form though pityriasiform, flexural and follicular lesions may also be present. Rarely, it may produce erythroderma.

Patient should be explained at the outset that there is no permanent cure, and the condition may require treatment for many years. Medicated shampoos containing selenium sulfide, ketoconazole, tar or 1% terbinafine may be used. Appropriate treatment of secondary bacterial infections also helps. Mild steroid ointments may be used for the acute forms.

For unresponsive cases, a course of UVB therapy, oral ketoconazole, or itraconazole may be used. Systemic steroids may be needed for generalized seborrhoeic dermatitis. Isotretinoin may also be helpful.

Lichen Planus

Lichen planus can be classically described as a disease with the following features:

- Plentiful polished.
- Pruritic.
- Purple.
- Polygonal.
- Papules.

Etiopathogenesis

- LP remains an idiopathic condition.
- Viral infection, autoimmune reaction, and psychogenic origin.
- Viral hepatitis, neurologic disease, severe psychic trauma, GVH.

Clinical Features

- Wickham's striae: White network on the surface of the papules.
- The characteristic oral findings in LP, are a white netlike or reticulated, patterned discoloration of the buccal mucosa or other oral mucosal surfaces. (Rerticulated, atrophic, popular, erosive, bullous, erosive, desquamitive gingivitis).
- Pruritus is typically intense in LP. Usually induces rubbing, rather than scratching, for relief.
- Nail changes occur in 10% of patients and include onychodystrophy (including "20-nail dystrophy") as well as the less severe manifestations of longitudinal ridging, irregular pitting,

nailplate splitting, nail loss, and pterygium formation.

Histopathologic Appearance of Lichen Planus

- The statum corneum is thickened (hyperkeratotic) with no retained keratinocytic nuclei (no parakeratosis).
- The granular layer is accentuated.
- The Malpighian layer is irregularly thickened, demonstrating **"sawtooth"** acanthosis and occasional necrotic keratinocytes.
- The basal layer is disrupted and appears lost or flattened.
- The dermal-epidermal junction is vacuolated and obscured by a band-like lymphocytic infiltrate which fills the upper dermis. The lymphocytic infiltrate is so typical of LP that any similar pattern is referred to as a "lichenoid infiltrate".

DIFFERENTIAL DIAGNOSIS OF AN LP-LIKE ERUPTION

LP-like drug eruptions are common and may indistinguishable from classic LP. Histopathogic clues are parakeratosis and eosinophil.

Twenty-nail Dystrophy

The etiology of twenty-nail dystrophy is controversial. This nail disorder affects mostly children and is not associated with cutaneous LP. It involves all 20 nails, showing excessive longitudinal ridging with thin, brittle, opalescent nails. Although some consider LP as a possible etiology, nail biopsy studies have shown a spongiotic inflammation and not a lichenoid process.

MULTIPLE CHOICE QUESTIONS

1. The drugs used in treatment of psoriasis are all *except*:
A. Methothexate
B. Coal tar
C. Retinoids
D. Systemic steroids

2. The mechanism of action of psoralin is:
A. Binding to DNA
B. Inhibiting protein synthesis
C. Inhibits angiogenosis
D. Inhibits peratinization

3. All of the following are histological features of psoriasis *except*:
A. Acanthosis
B. Parakeratosis
C. Monro's michoalescess
D. Colloid bodies

4. Impetigo herptiformis is:
A. Grouped lesions of impetigo seen in children
B. Pustular psoriasis in pregnancy
C. Other name for bulbous impetigo
D. A type of herpes virus infections

5. Nail changes in lichen planus are all *except*:
A. Pteryguim
B. Pitting
C. Thing of nail plate
D. Oil drop sign

6. Intra-epidermal micro-alescesses are seen in all *except*:
A. Psoriasis
B. Mycrosis fungoides
C. Peiters syndrome
D. Lichen planus

7. On histopathology "Ball in clutch" appearance is described in:
A. Pithriasis rubra pilasis
B. Lichen nitidies
C. Lichen amycoidosis
D. Discoid lupus erythematosis

8. The short contact therapy in psoriasis can be done with:
A. Topical corticosteroids
B. Dithranol
C. Coal tar
D. Any of the above

9. Which of the following histopathological features is not diagnostic of psoriasis?
A. Munro's microabscesses
B. Spongiform pustule of Kogoj
C. Koilocytosis
D. Extensive parakeratosis

10. Auspitz sign in psoriasis is taken as positive when:
A. Fine bleeding point seen on scales removal
B. Thin transparent membrane seen on scales removal
C. Easy removal of scales
D. Lesions at the site of trauma

11. Twenty nail dystrophy is associated with all *except*:
A. Lichen planus
B. Psoriasis
C. Alopecia areata
D. Pemphigus

1 D 2 A 3 D 4 B 5 D 6 D 7 B 8 B 9 C 10 A 11 D

12. Civatte bodies (colloid bodies) are seen in:
A. Pemphigus
B. Lichen planus
C. Herpes zoster
D. Epidermolysis bullosa

13. Calcanean spur on X-ray is characteristic of:
A. Reiter's disease
B. Psoriatic arthritis
C. Ankylosing spondylitis
D. Bechet's disease

14. Berkeley's membrane is seen in:
A. Pemphigus
B. Psoriasis
C. Pityriasis rosea
D. Pemphigoid

15. Following are true of psoriatic arthritis *except:*
A. Destructive arthritics
B. Rheumatoid factor absent
C. Distal interphalangeal joints affected
D. Mono-articular

16. Tar preparations used in treating psoriasis act by:
A. Cytotoxic
B. Immunosuppression
C. Anti-inflammatory
D. All of the above

17. Skin and kidney may be affected by the same pathological process in the following disease *except*:
A. Angiokeratoma corporis diffusum
B. Psoriasis
C. Neurofibromatosis
D. Systemic lupus erythematous

18. The turnover time of epidermis in psoriasis is:
A. 4 days
B. 8 days
C. 14 days
D. 28 days

19. Psoriasiform lesions are seen in:
A. Glucagonoma
B. Reiter's syndrome
C. Mycosis fungoides
D. All of the above

20. Following are true of psoriasis *except*:
A. Genetically determined
B. Scaling red patches
C. Affects 1-2% population
D. Koebenerization
E. Commonly flexor aspects

21. Pustular psoriasis most commonly affects:
A. Palnus and soles
B. Scalp
C. Trunk
D. Limbs

22. Psoriasis is exacerbated by:
A. Lithium
B. Beta-blockers
C. Antimalarials
D. All of the above

23. The active component of Lassar's paste is:
A. Zinc oxide
B. Dithranol
C. Coal tar
D. Steroids

24. Topical steroids can be used in psoriasis involving the following areas *except*:
A. Face
B. Palms and soles
C. Scalp
D. Trunk

12 B 13 A 14 B 15 D 16 D 17 B 18 A 19 D 20 E 21 A 22 D
23 A 24 D

25. Dose of 8-methoxy psoralin is:
- **A.** 0.6 mg/kg
- **B.** 6 mg/kg
- **C.** 10-12 mg/kg
- **D.** 1 mg/kg

26. Drug of choice for pustular psoriasis is:
- **A.** Oral retinoids
- **B.** PUVA
- **C.** Methotrexate
- **D.** Steroids

27. Herald patch is seen in:
- **A.** Prosea
- **B.** Psoriasis
- **C.** Lichen planus
- **D.** Leprosy

28. Which of the following is pruritic?
- **A.** Lichen planus
- **B.** Secondary syphilis rash
- **C.** Tinea versicolar
- **D.** Ichthosis

29. Woronoff's ring is implied to be caused due to abnormal levels of:
- **A.** Leukothenes
- **B.** Prostaglandin's
- **C.** Histamine
- **D.** Serotonin

30. A 30-year-old male presents with pruritic flat-topped papules on his forearm and a white lacework pattern in the buccal mucosa. Most likely diagnosis is:
- **A.** Psoriasis
- **B.** Lichen planus
- **C.** P. rosea
- **D.** Hansen's disease

31. Pseudopelade is characteristically seen in:
- **A.** Alopecia areata
- **B.** Lichen planus
- **C.** Psoriasis
- **D.** Tinea capitis

32. All are true of lichen planus *except*:
- **A.** Wickham's strial
- **B.** Shing violaceous flat topped polygonal papules
- **C.** Pruritic
- **D.** Basal cell degeneration seen on histopathology
- **E.** Auspitz sign is positive

33. Acneiform eruptions are seen with all *except*:
- **A.** Steroids
- **B.** Bromides and iodides
- **C.** INH
- **D.** OCP_S
- **E.** Rifampicin

34. Koebner's phenomenon is not seen in
- **A.** Psoriasis vulgaris
- **B.** Lichen planus
- **C.** Basal cell carcinoma
- **D.** Verruca plana

35. Auspitz sign is positive in:
- **A.** Ichthyosis vulgaris
- **B.** Warts
- **C.** Psoriasis vulgaris
- **D.** Urticaria pigmentosa

36. Kobner's phenomenon is seen in:
- **A.** Lichen planus
- **B.** Psoriasis vulgaris
- **C.** Warts
- **D.** All of the above

---

25 A **26 D** **27 A** **28 A** **29 B** **30 B** **31 B** **32 E** **33 E** **34 C** **35 C** **36 D**

37. PUVA therapy can be used to treat:
A. Psoriasis
B. Atopic dermatitis
C. Alopecia areata
D. Vitiligo
E. All of the above

38. Pitting of nails is characteristic of:
A. Psoriasis
B. Warts
C. Ring worm infection
D. Iron deficiency anaemia

39. Goeckerman's regimen is used in treatment of:
A. Acne vulgaris
B. Psoriasis vulgaris
C. Pitryriasis rubra pitaris
D. Erythroderma

40. Ingram's regimen all are true *except*:
A. Treatment modality for psoriasis
B. Includes application of dithranol
C. Patient is exposed to UVB
D. Patient is exposed to UVA

41. The anti histamine which might cause exacerbation of psoriasis:
A. Cetrizine
B. Clemestine
C. Diphenhydramine
D. Terfenadine

42. Effectiveness of methotrexate in psoriasis is apparently due to its effect on which phase of cell-cycle:
A. M
B. S
C. G_1
D. G_2

43. Pityrosporum orbiculare (causing Tinea versicolor) causes hypopigmentation of skin due to:
A. Direct damage to melanocytes
B. Utilization of substrate DOPA by the yeast
C. Production of azelaic acid which inhibits melanocyte tyrosinase
D. Inhibition of melamosome transfer

44. Tazarotene is used in the treatment of:
A. Alopecia areata
B. Lichen planus
C. Psoriasis
D. Herpes zoster

45. The pathogenesis of nail pits in psoriasis is:
A. Punctate defects in the cuticle
B. Secondary effects of proximal nail fold psoriasis
C. Punctate parakeratosis in the proximal matrix
D. Capillary haemorrhage in the proximal latrix
E. None of the above

37 E 38 A 39 B 40 D 41 D 42 B 43 C 44 C 45 C

Chapter 4

Vesiculobullous Disorders

Classification of blisters

Classification of Intra-epidermal Blisters	*Dermal-Epidermal Junction*
Granular layer • Friction blister • Pemphigus foliaceus • Subcorneal pustular dermatosis • Staphylococcal scalded-skin syndrome • Bullous impetigo *Spinous layer* • Eczematous dermatitis • Herpes virus infection • Familial benign pemphigus *Suprabasal* • Pemphigus vulgaris • Darier's disease *Basal layer* • Erythema multiforme • Lupus erythematosus • Lichen planus • Epidermolysis bullosa simplex	*Junctional (at the lamina lucida)* • Junctional epidermolysis bullosa • Bullous pemphigoid *Dermolytic (below basal lamina)* • Epidermolysis bullosa dystrophicans • Epidermolysis bullosa acquisita • Porphyria cutanea tarda • Dermatitis herpetiformis

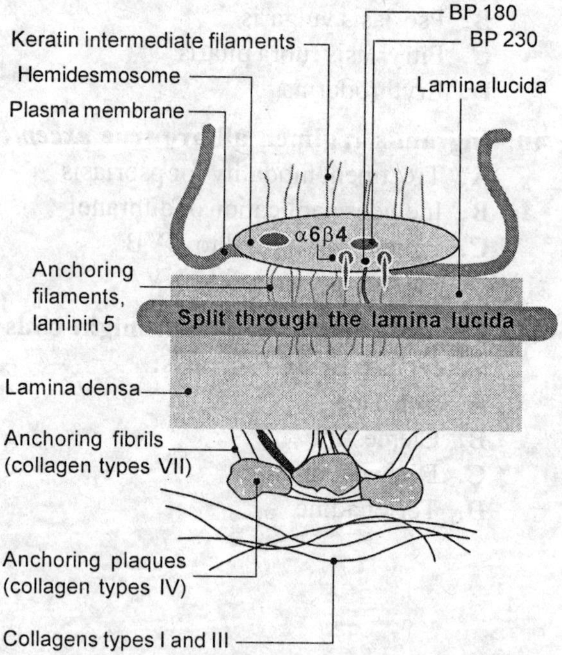

Fig. 4.1: Molecular structure of the hemidesmosome and the basement membrane zone of the epidermis

Non-immune (Epidermolysis Bullosa)

Acquired autoimmune blistering disorders (pemphigus, bullous pemphigoid, dermatitis herpetiformis, chronic bullous dermatosis of childhood, epidermolysis bullosa acquisita).

Epidermolysis Bullosa

- Epidermolysis bullosa (EB) comprises a group of genetically determined skin disorders characterized by blistering of the skin and mucosae at birth or soon afterwards, following mild

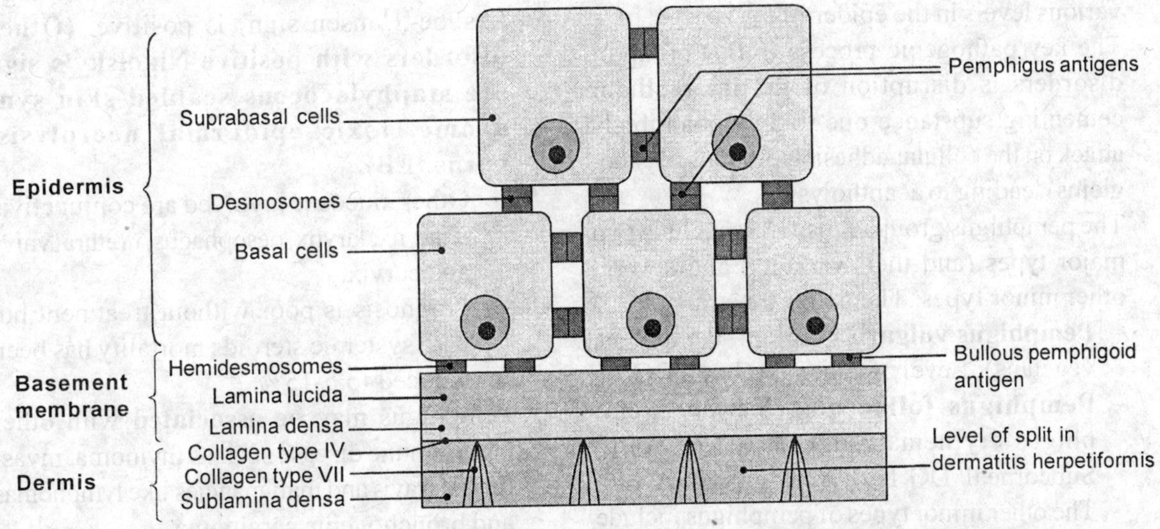

Fig. 14.2: Structure of the epidermis and sites of target antigens/cleavage in bullous diseases

mechanical trauma (due to increased fragility of skin). Thus an alternative term for these disorders could be the 'mechanobullous' disorders.

- There are three main types of EB are:
  - EB simplex (intraepidermal).
  - Junctional EB (split through the basement membrane zone).
  - Dystrophic EB (split in the subepidermal level).
- EB simplex is the most common and mildest form of EB of autosomal dominant inheritance. It is characterized by onset of blistering over trauma prone sites at birth or infancy. Lesions heat without scarring. Mucosae, nails and hair are essentially uninvolved.
- Junctional EB are autosomal recessive disorders and are broadly classified into two main types, the lethal and non-lethal forms. They present at birth or soon after with severe fragility of the skin leading to extensive blistering and denudation. Oropharyngeal mucosae may be severely involved. Teeth may be malformed and prematurely lost and nails may be shed. This is the most fatal type of EB.
- Dystrophic EB is characterized by skin fragility, scarring **with milia nail changes and** have either autosomal recessive or dominant inheritance. The most severe autosomal recessive form is characterized by:
  - Oral blisters and scarring leading to ankyloglossia.
  - Oesophageal lesions causing painful dysphagia and later oesophageal strictures.
  - Perianal blistering, erosions and scarring causing stenosis and fecal retention.
  - Ocular complication–symblepharon, corneal erosions and opacity.
  - Repeated blistetring and progressive scarring—contractures and deformities (e.g. **'Mitten hands'**).
- Gene therapy appears as a realistic goal in the future.
- Some drugs have been tried–Phenytoin, retinoids, Vit E and steroids.

Pemphigus

- Pemphigus is derived from the Greek 'pemphix' meaning blister or bubble and is characterized by intraepidermal blistering at various levels in the epidermis.

- The key pathogenic process in this group of disorders is disruption of the intercellular cementing substance due to an autoantibody attack on the cellular adhesion proteins (desmogleins) leading to acantholysis.
- The pemphigus group of disorders include two major types (and their variants) and several other minor types. The major types are:
  - **Pemphigus vulgaris** (Variant–Pemphigus vegetans): Level of split suprabasal DG3.
  - **Pemphigus foliaceous** (Variant–Pemphigus erythematosus): Level of split–Subcorneal DG 1.
  - The other minor types of pemphigus include paraneoplastic pemphigus, drug induced pemphigus, IgA pemphigus and neonatal pemphigus.

Pemphigus Vulgaris

- Most common form of pemphigus, accounting for up to 80% of pemphigus cases. Occurs at any age, most commonly between fourth– sixth decades. In India, it occurs at younger age.
- It is due IgG antibodies directed against epidermal cell adhesion molecules (desmoglein 3)–disruption of intercellular cementing substance–loss of adhesion between epidermal cells (acantholysis)–intraepidermal blistering.
- **Clinical features:**
  - Almost all patients have **mucosal lesions, 50-70%** present with painful oral erosions. Lesions may be limited to oral cavity for months to one year.
  - Skin–flaccid bullae on normal or erythematous skin, with a predilection for scalp, face, trunk, axillae and groins and pressure sites. Bullae rupture producing painful erosions that show no tendency to heal spontaneously.
- Nikolsky's sign and Bulla spread sign (Asboe–Hansen sign) is positive. **(Other disorders with positive Nikolsky's sign are staphylococcus scabled skin syndrome, toxic epidermal necrolysis, burns, EB).**
  - Other mucosae involved are conjunctiva, pharynx, larynx, oesophagus, urethra, vulva and cervix.
  - Prognosis is poor without treatment but with systemic steroids mortality has been reduced to 5-15%.
- Pemphigus may **be associated** with other autoimmune disease such as thymoma, myasthenia gravis and malignancies like lymphomas and bronchogenic carcinoma.
- **Diagnosis**
  - **Tzanck** smear from the floor of the blister shows acantholytic cells. **Acantholytic** cell is a large, rounded epidermal cell with a large nucleus, perinuclear halo and peripheral condensation of cytoplasm
  - Histopathological examination of a blister shows a supra–basal cleft in the epidermis. The basal keratinocytes remain attached to the basement membrane but are separated form each other and stand like a **'row of tombstones'**.
  - Immunofluorescence studies are the gold standard in diagnosis of the autoimmune blistering disorders. In pemphigus vulgaris, direct immunofluorescence done on the lesional skin shows deposition of intercellular IgG throughout the epidermis in a **'fish-net' pattern**. Indirect immunofluorescence done to determine levels of pathogenic antibodies in the sera of the patients shows circulating intercellular IgG antibodies in 80-90% of the cases. Levels of these antibodies correlate with disease activity.

Pemphigus Foliaceous

- This disorder, characterized by blistering at a higher level in the epidermis is less common than pemphigus vulgaris and accounts for only15-20% of pemphigus cases.
- It is caused by IgG antibodies directed against intercellular adhesion disruption of intercellular cementing substance of upper epidermal cells—subcorenal blister formation.
- Pemphigus erythematosus is variant of pemphigus foliaceous characterized by immunological features of both pemphigus and lupus erythematosus (LE), that is, intercellular IgG C3 in the epidermis (as in pemphigus) and in the basement membrane zone (as in LE) and antinuclear antibodies (as in LE). Clinically, erythematous, scarly rash over the nose and cheeks simulate LE while lesions on the trunk are similar to those in pemphigus foliaceous
- *Treatment:* Steroids, also tetracycline's and niacinamide.

Other Variants of Pemphigus

- Endemic pemphigus foliaceous (Fogo Selvagem) is a variant of pemphigus foliaceous, endemic to certain parts of South America and is postulated to be precipitated by bites of **the black fly *(Simulum simulidae).*** The burnt appearance and burning sensation gave the disease its name, fogo selvagen, meaning "wild fire".
- Drug induced **pemphigus (penicillamine, captropril, pyritinol, penicillin, rifampicin)** –clinically commonly present as pemphigus foliaceous.
- Paranoplastic pemphigus–a polymorphous blistering eruption with mucocutaneous ulcerations having an underlying neoplasm.
- Pemphigus herpetiformis–superficial vesicles and inflammatory papules occur in herpetiform distribution.
- IgA pemphigus–has bound and circulating IgA autoantibodies against intraepidermal cell surface antigens and clinically may resemble subcorneal pustular dermatosis.
- Juvenile pemphigus—pemphigus occurring before 20 years of age.
- Neonatal pemphigus–due to transplacental transfer of maternal anti-intercellular cement substance antibodies to the fetus. Blisters resolves in 2 weeks.

Treatment of Pemphigus

- The mainstay of therapy in the pemphigus group of disorders is with systemic steroids, which can be given as conventional therapy (oral prednisolone in the dose of 1 mg per kg body weight) or as pulse therapy. An upcoming mode of therapy is the dexamethasone cyclophosphamide pulse regimen consisting of 100 mg or IV dexamethasone in 5% dextrose intrusion on 3 consecutive days of each of month combined with IV cyclophosphamide 500 mg bolus dose on day 1 of the pulse and oral cyclophosphamide 50 mg on other days. This therapy reduce the conventional side effects of steroids.
- The other modalities of therapy include adjuvant therapy with dapsone, azathioprine, cyclosporine, methotrexate, gold salts and plasmapheresis and are essentially to reduce the side effects or to control the severe form of pemphigus.

Bullous Pemphigoid (BP)

- Onset usually after 60 years of age.
- Basic pathogenic process is due to IgG antibodies against components of the basement membrane zone (BMZ–structure which binds epidermis to the underlying dermis and mesenchyme)–loss of structural integrity of the BMZ due to resultant inflammation – separation of the intact epidermis from underlying dermis–**subepidermal cleft formation.**

- **Clinical Features:**
  - Proceeded by **pruritus with or without urticarial wheals** lasting usually for 1-3 weeks.
  - **Tense bullae** on normal or erythematous skin predominantly over flexural aspects of the limbs, lower abdomen, groins and axillae. Facial skin and scalp relatively spared.
  - Lesions rupture to leave erosions that heal spontaneously with postinflammatory hyperpigmentation.
  - Nikolsky's sign usually negative; Bulla spread sign +/-.
  - Mucosal lesions rare and less severe than in pemphigus vulgaris and almost nerve the presenting features.
- Bullous pemphigoid may be associated with an underlying malignancy (gastric carcinoma commonly) and may be associated with diabetes mellitus, rheumatoid arthritis psoriasis.

Diagnosis

- **Direct immunofluorescence** of perilesional skin shows linear IgG (45–90%) and C3 (80–100%) deposition in the basement membrane zone. Indirect immunofluorescence studies done on the patient's sera show circulating IgG autoantibodies in most cases but unlike in pemphigus, their titers do not correlate with disease activity.
- Prognosis of bullous pemphigoid is better than pemphigus and it runs a chronic self-limiting course. It may be fatal in the active stage in the elderly or debilitated patients.

Treatment

- The mainstay of treatment is a topical or systemic steroid.

  Cicatricial pemphigoid. Sequelae include oropharyngeal adhesions, oesophageal strictures, stridor, introital shrinkage, symblepharon and 'statue eye'. Unlike bullous pemphigoid, this disorder is not self-limiting and has a chronic debilitating course.

- **Herpes gestationis** pregnancy (21-28 weeks of gestation) or within 1st week postanatally. Clinically the disease starts as severe pruritus with urticarial wheals and plaques followed by blistering predominantly in the periumbilical area, lower abdomen and thighs. Mucosal involvement is rare and lesions improve postpartum. Recurrence may occur in subsequent pregnancies, premenstrually or with oral contraceptive pills (OCPs). Direct immunofluorescence shows linear **C3** deposits at the BMZ with IgG in some cases.

To differentiate between the subepidermal disorders–salt split analysis–A split at the level of lamina lucida.

Roof—BP, HG.

Base—EB acquisita, CP, Linear IgA, CBDC.

Characteristic Pemphigoid	*Bullous vulgaris*	*Pemphigus*
Age	> 60 years	Middle age
Pruritus	++	Not present
Blister	Tense	Flaccid
Sites	Flexures, groins; axillae abdomen	Face, scalp, trunk, pressure points
Erosion	Spontaneously heal	Extend peripherally
Nikolsk's sign	Negative	Positive
Oral lesions	40% less severe Almost never a presenting feature	80-90% severe Commonly the presenting symptom
Prognosis	Benign, self-limiting	Poor without treatment

Dermatitis Herpetiformis (DH)

- DH is defined as an intensely pruritic, chronic, recurrent, papulovesicular disease with an underlying gluten-sensitive enteropathy which may be asymptomatic.
- **Clinical Features:**
  - Onset at any age, usually between 20-55 years of age.
  - Males outnumber females.
  - **Pruritus** is the first and predominant symptom followed by a symmetrical erup-

tion of erythematous papules and papulo-vesicles, which are so rapidly excoriated that intact vesicles are difficult to demonstrate.

- **Sites**–extensor aspects of limbs (elbows and knees), buttocks, natal cleft, shoulder upper back, face and scalp. Grouping of lesions accounts for it being described as herpetiformis (not associated with herpes virus).
- Oral lesions are common but asymptomatic.
- Provocation of lesions occurs with iodides orally or in iodide patch testing.
- Histologically examination best done on lesions that have not blistered or ruptured and reveals neutrophilic microabscess at the tips of dermal papillae.
- Direct immunofluorescence is the most reliable diagnostic criterion and should be performed on clinically normal skin (preferably of the buttocks). It reveals **granular IgA deposits in dermal papillae.**
- Indirect immunofluorescence is negative for anti–BMZ or dermal autoantibodies but antithyroid and antigliadin antibodies may be seen.

• **Treatment**

- Dapsone 100-200 mg/day (upto 400 mg/day) is the drug of choice.
- Strict adherence to a gluten-free diet for prolonged periods (e.g. 6 to 12 months) may control the disease in some patients, obviating of reducing the requirement for drug therapy.
- Avoid–wheat barley rye.
- Take—RMO **(rice, maize, oats).**

Chronic Bullous Dermatoses of Childhood (CBDC)

- CBDC is defined as a chronic acquired autoimmune subepidermal blistering disease of children characterized by IgA BMZ antibodies.
- Onset is usually at around 5 years of age (toddlers and preschool children).
- Uriticarial plaques with blistering at the edges –**'string of pearls'** appearance and localization of lesions **around orifices** (perioral, perigenital).
- Spontaneous remission usually occurs with age.
- Direct immunofluorescence shows linear IgA at BMZ.
- Dapsone is usually effective, and may be combined with low dose steroids in refractory cases.

TIPS

1. **Acantholysis:**
   - *Primary*–Pemphigus, Darier's diseases, Grover's, Hailey-Hailey diseases.
   - *Secondary*–Herpes, SCC, trauma, burns.
   - *IgA disorders*–DH, IgA pemphigus, CBDC, Linear IgA disease.
2. **Non-immune disorders:**
   - SCPD, Grover's, Darier's diseases, EB acq.
3. **Split:**
   - *Subcorneal:* FCI (P foliaceous, SCPD, Impetigo).
   - *Intraepidermal:* Herpes.
   - *Suprabasal:* P Vulgaris, Hailey-Hailey disease, Darier's.
   - *Sub epidermal:* BEDC (BP, EB, DH, CP, CBDC).

Disorders	*Site of split*	*Pathogenic antibody*
P. vulgaris	Suprabasal	IgG
P. foliaceous/erythematosus	Subcorneal	IgG
Paraneoplastic pemphigus	Suprabasal	IgG
BP/HG/CP	Subepidermal	IgG & C3
EBA	Subepidermal	IgG
Dermatitis herpetiformis	Subepidermal	IgG
CBDC	Subepidermal	IgG

- (**Note:** Epidermolysis bullosa are a group of genetic disorders with structural defects but no autoantibodies).

Epidermolysis Bullosa Acquistia (EBA)

- It is defined as a chronic, acquired autoimmune blistering disorder characterized either by trauma-induced subepidermal blistering or with a clinical picture in distinguishable from bullous pemphigoid.
- IgG class of autoantibodies directed against collagen VII causes it. Collagen VII is the major component of the anchoring fibrils found in the subepidermal zone (differentiate from hereditary epidermolysis bullosa dystrophica in which there is a collagen VII structural defect leading to reduced or absent collagen VII in the anchoring fibrils).
- Clinically this presents in two forms:
  - Mechanobullous type—blistering over trauma prone sites, which heals with scarring and milia formation; nails may be dystrophic.
  - Bullous pemphigoid (BP) like—mimics bullous pemphigoid and has a better prognosis.
- Mucosal lesions may be present in a variable number of patients.
- Histology shows subepidermal cleft with neutrophilic infiltrate in the BP type while sparse inflammatory infiltrate in the mechanobullous type.
- Direct immunofluorescence on perilesional skin shows thick polyclonal band of deposition of IgG and C3 and sometimes IgA and IgM in the BMZ.
- Steroids in combination with dapsone or adjuvant immunosuppressive are the usual line of therapy. The mechanobullous type is resistant to most modalities of treatment.

Vesiculobullous disorders of skin (III)

	Pemphigus	*Pemphigoid*	*Linear IgA dermatosis*	*Herpes gestationis*	*Chronic bullous disease of childhood*	*Dermatitis herpetiformis*
Age of onset	4th-5th decade (30-50y)	6th to 8th decade (50-80 y)	Middle age	Pregnant women	1st decade of life	3rd decade (20-30y)
HLA association	HLA-AIO, A26 and DRW_4 (especially in jews)	NIL	NIL	NIL	HLA-Bm8	HLA-B_8, DRW-3
Clinical features	Discrete, flaccid bullae arising over apparently normal skin. Nikolsky and bulla spread signs are (+). Involves scalp, chest, back, inter-triginous areas	Tense bullae arising over erythematous and/or urticarial plaques. Localized on the flexures, Nikolsky and bulla signs are negative	Blisters smaller than pemphigoid but larger than DH. Localize in flexural areas	Erythematous oedematous papulo-vesicles and plaques and/ or large tense bullae. Lesions may be grouped or coalesce. Abdomen, palms, soles, chest, and face usually involved	Grouped, tense vesicles and/or bullae. 'Cluster of jewel' pattern. Localize on the flexures and pelvic region	Vesicles and/or papulovesicles 3-6 mm in size. Distributed symmetrically over extensor surfaces. Elbows, proximal forearms, knees, buttocks and sacrum
Mucosal involvement	Involved in almost all cases. May precede and/or accompany cutaneous lesions	Oral lesions seen only in 20% cases. Involvement of other mucosae uncommon	Infrequent	Mucosae spared	Mucosae spared	Mucosae spared

Contd...

Contd...

	Pemphigus	*Pemphigoid*	*Linear IgA dermatosis*	*Herpes gestationis*	*Chronic bullous disease of childhood*	*Dermatitis herpetiformis*
	(Oropharyngeal, genital, nasal mucosal involved commonly)					
Variants	Pemphigus vulgaris + vegitans. Pemphigus foliaceous and Pemphigus erythematous. Herpetiform, neonatal, drug induced	Classical bullous localized nodular, vesicular, childhood variant	NIL	NIL	NIL	NIL
Associated features	NIL	NIL	NIL	NIL	NIL	Gluten sensitive enteropathy
Precipitating factors	Drugs like D-penicillamine, rifampicin, piroxicam, phenytoin, captopril, phenobarbitone	NIL	NIL	Pregnancy usually 2nd and 3rd trimester At times flares up during postpartum period	NIL	Ingestion of gluten containing diet. Also iodine
Location of blister (on histopathology)	Intra-epidermal suprabasal in PV. Subcutaneous in PF	Sub-epidermal in the lamina lucida of BMZ	Sub-epidermal in lamina lucida of BMZ	Sub-epidermal in the lamina lucida of BMZ	Sub-epidermal in lamina lucida of BMZ	Sub-epidermal at the tips of dermal papular
Direct immunofluorescence	Deposition of IgG and C_3 in the intercellular spares	Linear deposition of IgG and C_3 at the lamina lucida of BMZ	Linear deposition of IgA at the lamina lucida of BMZ or below BMZ	Linear deposition of C_3 at the lamina lucida of BMZ. 30% also show deposits of IgG at the same site	Linear deposition of IgA at the lamina lucida of BMZ	Granular deposits of IgA at the tips of dermal papillae of uninvolved skin
Indirect immunofluorescence	IgG pemphigus antibodies in the serum. Titres directly proportional to severity of disease	Serum IgG anti-BNZ antibodies in 90% cases	Negative	Serum IgG anti-BNZ antibodies in 10-20% cases	Circulating IgA anti-BNZ antibodies	Negative
Treatment	High dose corticosteroids. Immuno-suppressive adjuvant	Moderately high doses of steroids. Immunosuppressive adjuvant	Dapsone alone or in combination with steroids	Corticosteroids	Dapsone	Dapsone

MULTIPLE CHOICE QUESTIONS

1. Nikolsky's sign is positive in:
A. TEN
B. Pemphigoid
C. Pemphigus
D. Staphylococcal scalded skin syndrome

2. For immunofluorescence test in patients with pemphigus or dermatitis herpetiformis the site for skin biopsy is:
A. Intact vesicle
B. Skin distant from the lesion
C. Perilesional skin
D. Deroofed vesicle

3. Split in pemphigoid is located at:
A. Stratum-granulosum
B. Suprabasal
C. Sub epidermal
D. Within the basement membrane

4. Treatment of dermatitis herpetiformis includes all *except*:
A. Dapsone
B. Potassium iodide
C. Sulphapyridine
D. Gluten free diet

5. All true of epidermolysis bullosa *except*:
A. Genetically determined
B. Characterised by blistering of the skin and mucosae resulting from minor mechanical trauma
C. Some forms can be lethal
D. Patients show dramatic improvement with systemic steroids
E. Treatment is largely symptomatic and unsatisfactory

6. The method of choice for diagnosing epidermolysis bullosa is:
A. Direct immunofluorescence
B. Indirect immunofluorescence using sodium chloride skin
C. Electron microscopy
D. Therapeutic trial with steroids

7. 'Mitten-hand' is seen in:
A. Epidermolysis bullosa simplex
B. Epidermolysis bullosa junctional
C. Epidermolysis bullosa dystrophica
D. Congenital localized absence of skin

8. Scarring of the skin and mucous membranes is seen with:
A. Benign mucosal pemphigoid
B. Pemphigus vulgaris
C. Epidermolysis bullosa acquisita
D. Pemphigus erythematosus

9. 'Row of tomb stones' appearance on histopathology is characteristic of:
A. Pemphigoid
B. Hailey-Hailey disease
C. Pemphigus vulgaris
D. Pemphigus foliaceous

10. Which of the following is the drug of first choice for Non-Gonococcal Urethritis?
A. Ceftriaxone
B. Ciprofloxacin
C. Doxycycline
D. Minocycline

1 C 2 C 3 D 4 B 5 D 6 C 7 B 8 A 9 C 10 C

11. A 30-year-old male had severely itchy papulo-vesicular lesions on extremities, knees, elbows and buttocks for one year. Direct immunofluorescence staining of the lesions showed IgA deposition at dermoepidermal junction. The most probable diagnosis is:
- A. Pemphigus vulgaris
- B. Bullous pemphigoid
- C. Dermatitis herpetiformis
- D. Nummular eczema

12. Intercellular antibody deposited in pemphigus vulgaris is:
- A. IgG
- B. IgA
- C. IgM
- D. Complement

13. Gluten enteropathy is a feature of:
- A. Pemphigus vulgaris
- B. Bullous pemphigoid
- C. Dermatitis herpetiformis
- D. Epidermolysis bullosa simplex

14. Match the following:

A. Acantholysis	i. Pemphigus
B. Balloon degeneration	ii. Contact dermatitis
C. Basal cell degeneration	iii. Herpes zoster
D. Spongiosis	iv. Darier's disease
E. Dysveratosis	v. Lichen planus

15. Acantholysis is seen in all *except*:
- A. Pemphigus
- B. Pemphigoid
- C. Herpes simplex
- D. Vaccinia

16. 'Cluster of Jewels' is seen clinically in:
- A. Chronic bullous dermatosis of childhood
- B. SSSS
- C. Impetigo
- D. Dermatitis herpetiformis

17. Integrins and cadherins are important in pathogenesis of:
- A. Pemphigus
- B. Psoriasis
- C. Lichen planus
- D. Pseudoxanthoma elasticum

18. All true of epidermolysis bullosa *except:*
- A. Genetically determined
- B. Characterised by blistering of the skin and mucosae resulting from minor mechanical trauma
- C. Some forms can be lethal
- D. Patients show dramatic improvement with systemic steroids
- E. Treatment is largely symptomatic and unsatisfactory

19. 60-year-old man presenting with tense bullae with no oral involvement diagnosis is:
- A. Pemphigus vulgaris
- B. Pemphigoid
- C. Pemphigus foliaceous
- D. Epidermolysis bullosa simplex

20. Most common cause of death in pemphigus:
- A. Secondary infections
- B. Electrolyle imbalance
- C. Hypothermia
- D. Cachexia

21. Deposit of IgA in papillary dermis are seen in:
- A. Pemphigus
- B. Linear IgA disease
- C. Dermatitis herpetiformis
- D. Herpes gestations

---

11 C 12 A 13 C 14 A(i), B(iii), C(v), D(ii), E(iv) 15 B 16 A 17 A 18 D 19 B
20 A 21 C

22. Mucous membranes are usually involved in:
A. Pemphigus vulgaris
B. Pemphigoid
C. Dermatitis herpetiformis
D. All of the above

23. Drug of choice for treating dermatitis herpetiformis:
A. Dapsone
B. Systemic steroids
C. Antihistamines
D. Cotrimoxazole

24. Oral retinoids are indicated in the treatment of all *except*:
A. Acne vulgaris
B. Psoriasis vulgaris
C. Darier's disease
D. Ichthysosis
E. Pemphigus vulgaris

25. Intraepidermal bulla is the feature of:
A. Pemphigoid
B. Pemphigus
C. Dermatitis herpetiformis
D. Herpes gestations

26. 60-year-old man presenting with tense bullae with no oral involvement diagnosis is:
A. Pemphigus vulgaris
B. Pemphigoid
C. Pemphigus foliaceous
D. Epidermolysis bullosa simplex

27. Pruritic vesiculobullous disorders of autoimmune aetiology–all *except*:
A. Pemphigus
B. Pemphigoid
C. Dermatitis herpetiformis
D. Linear IgA disease

28. Fogo salvagum closely resembles:
A. Pemphigus vulgaris
B. Pemphigus foliaceous
C. Pemphigus erythematosus
D. Paraneoplastic pemphigus

29. Dapsone is treatment of choice in:
A. Darier's disease
B. Ritter's disease
C. Dhuring's Broce disease
D. Schamberg disease

30. Cell detachment leading to acantholysis in Darier's disease is due to:
A. Autoantibodies directed against desmosomal components
B. Proteolysis of desmosomal proteins
C. Intercellular oedema
D. Intracellular oedema

31. Benign mucosal pemphigoid of head and neck area most often seen in middle aged males is called:
A. Burn's syndrome
B. Brunstig and Perry syndrome
C. Burger Grutz syndrome
D. Carpenter syndrome

22 A 23 A 24 E 25 B 26 B 27 A 28 B 29 C 30 B 31 B

Chapter 5

Connective Tissue Disorders

Connective disorders are multisystem disorder with prominent cutaneous manifestation. They are systemic lupus erythematosus, systemic sclerosis, dermatomyosistis, overlap—syndrome and mixed connective tissue disease.

Lupus Erythematosus

Lupus erythematosus is a multisystem disease of unknown origin characterized by the production of numerous diverse types of autoanti-bodies. Lupus erythematosus have wide spectum of manifestations ranging from solitary chronic skin lesions in chronic discoid lupus erythematosus (DLE) to widespread polymorphous lesions in subacute lupus erythematosus (SCLE) to multiple organ involvement in systemic lupus erythematosus (SLE).

GILLIAMS CLASSIFICATION

i. LE SPECIFIC

Acute Le—Malar trash, Ac exanthermata.
Subacute Le—Annular, papulosquamous.
Chronic Le.

ii. LE NON-SPECIFIC

Discoid Lupus Erythematosus (DLE)

- Most common form of cutaneous lupus erythematosus.
- Characterized by discrete, discoid, well-defined erythematous plaques covered with adherent scales. The lesions slowly expand with active inflammation at the periphery, leaving depressed scars, talangiectasis and permanent depigmentation.
- The central scarring with atrophy is very characteristic.
- These lesions occur most often on the face, scalp, ears or neck.
- Peeling the scale reveals and undersurface that looks like a carpet penetrated by several carpet tacks called **"carpet tack sign".**
- Scarring alopecia occurs in 60% of the cases.

Types

- Localized DLE: lesions occur only on the head or neck.
- Generalized DLE: lesions are seen both above and below the neck.

Prognosis

- DLE has a chronic progressive course. Patients with hematological and serological abnormalities have 6.5% risk of developing over SLE.
- The risk is higher in patients with disseminated DLE (22%).

Diagnosis

- Based on clinical features and histopathology.
- **Most sensitive tool is lupus band test in involved skin.**
- **Other tools: Eosinophilia, ANA, ssDNA.**

Histopathology

Characteristic histopathological changes are:
- Hyperkeratosis with follicular plugging.
- Irregular atrophy of the stratum malphighi.
- Liquefactive degeneration of the basal cell layer.
- Patchy perivascular and periappendigeal lymphocytic infiltration.
- Lupus band test—Direct immunofluorescence—positive after 6 weeks.

Treatment

- Photoprotection and topical sun screens.
- Topical or intralesional steroids or systemic corticosteroids.
- Chloroquine.

CLINICAL POINTS (FACE, DISCOID PATCH, PHOTOSENSITIVITY)

- **Most common type going into SLE—Lupus panniculitis.**
- **Mimic of breast cancer—Lupus panniculitis.**
- **Type with no surface changes—Tumid LE.**
- **Antibody specific for DLE ds DNA.**
- **Most sensitive tool for assessing progression to SLE-Lupus band test in normal skin.**

Subacute Lupus Erythematosus (SCLE)

- Characterized by scaly papules on the shoulders, extensor surfaces of the upper extremities, upper chest, upper back and neck in widespread and symmetric fashion.
- Above lesions evolve into two morphological types either into papulosquamous or annular and polycyclic lesions.
- All patients with SCLE have mild systemic complaints and 50% of the patients fulfil the criteria for the diagnosis of SLE.
- SCLE patients have antibodies to the cellular antigens **<u>Ro/SS-A and La/SS-B.</u>**
- **Neonatal LE—same antibody and clinical pattern—Heart block can be seen.**

Risk Factors of CCLE for Dissemination and/or Systemic Involvement

No single data can accurately predict which patient will have progressive skin disease or internal organ involvement. However, the following history or test results, in different combinations at appropriate settings, should alert the clinicians for close monitoring.

1. *Clinical:* Unexplained persistent fever, Raynaud's phenomenon, arthralgia/arthritis, diffuse alopecia, progressive lower limb oedema, mucocutaneous vasculitis, and CCLE affecting a very young patient.
2. *Laboratory tests:* Anaemia, thrombocytopenia, leucopenia and raised ESR.
   - Positive Anti-dsDNA and/or anti-Sm.
   - Very high ANA titre (some believed a correlation exists with dissemination of skin lesions. It is not a useful indicator of progression to SLE).
   - High titre of ACL.
   - Biological false positive test for syphilis.
   - Low titres of C3, C4.
3. *Lupus band test:* Deposits of IgG, IgM, IgA or all three in nonlesional, non-facial, sun protected skin is highly suggestive of SLE.
4. *Other:* HLA-B8 females at the ages of 15-40.

Systemic Lupus Erythematosus (SLE)

SLE is a multisystem disorder primarily affects skin, joints and vascular system. The age of onset is usually between 16 and 42 years occurring more frequently in females (F : M :: 8 : 1).

Etiology

- Exact cause is unknown but there is evidence to suggest the role of genetic, immune and various environmental factors.

- It has been postulated that four or more genes are involved in predisposing an individual to SLE.

The 1982 revised criteria for diagnosis of SLE are:

1. Malar rash.
2. Discoid rash.
3. Photosensitivity.
4. Oral or nasophageal ulceration.
5. Arthritis—nonerosive or two or more peripheral joints.
6. Serositis: Pleuritis or pericarditis.
7. Renal disorders: Persistent proteinuria (> 0.5 gm/day or > 3+), cellular casts (RBC, granular, tubular or mixed).
8. Neurological disorders: Seizure or psychosis.
9. Haematological disorders: Hemolytic anemia with reticulocytosis or Leukopenia (<4000/mm^3 on two or more occasions), or Lymphopenia (<1500/mm^3 on two or more occasions) or Thrombocytopenia (<1,00,000/mm^3).
10. Immunological disorder; Positive LE cell phenomenon, or Anti-DNA: Antibody to native DNA (nDNA) in abnormal titer, or Anti-Sm: Presence of antibody to Sm nuclear antigen or False positive serologic test for syphilis for at least six months and confirmed by TPI or FTA–ABS test.
11. ANA.

NOTE: A patient is said to have SLE if four or more criteria are satisfied, serially or simultaneously.

Chief Cutaneous Features

- Butterfly rash.
- Photosensitivity **(MC sign).**
- Raynaud's phenomenon.
- Non-scarring alopecia.
- Urticarial vasculitis.
- Mouth ulceration **(reticular pattern).**
- Chronic discoid LE lesion.
- Cutaneous vasculitis.

Investigation

- Lupus band test.
- C3, C4, CH50 levels.
- ANA (Most common pattern is **homogeneous;** peripheral pattern predictor of renal involvement).
- ds DNA.
- Antibodies—SSA (Ro), SSB (La), Sm, nRNP.

Treatment

SLE with only cutaneous lesions and arthritis:

- Photoprotection.
- NSAIDs, Antimalarials, prednisolone.
- Severe disease with end-organ prednisolone
  - Steroid pulse therapy.
  - Immunosuppressants such as azathioprine, cyclophosphamide methotrexate, chlorambucil and cyclosporine.

Scleroderma

Scleroderma (Gr. Skleros—hard and derma—skin) is a connective tissue disorder characterized by thickening and fibrosis of the skin.

Types

Circumscribed

- Morphea.

Systemic

- Progressive systemic sclerosis.
- CREST syndrome (Thibierge–Weissenbach syndrome).

Morphea

Localised morphea.

- Most common form of morphea.
- Occurs most commonly in females than males and primarily in young adults.
- Seen commonly on the trunk.
- These lesions of morphea may begin as erythematous macule, evolve into ivory-colored centers and violaceous bordered plaque.
- Lesions slowly involute over 3 to 5 years period leaving permanent atrophic skin or normal appearing skin behind.

Generalized morphea

- Lesions are more numerous and larger.
- Often coalesce to involve extensive portions of the body.
- Muscle atrophy may be associated.

Pansclerotic morphea (morphea profunda)

- Sclerosis involves dermis, panniculus, fascia, muscle and bones.
- There is disabling limitation of the joints.

En coup de sabre

- It is variant of linear scleroderma involving scalp parasagittally on frontal scalp and forehead.
- Often has the configuration of the stroke of a saber (en coup de sabre).

Treatment

- Topical steroid, intralesional steroids and chloroquine.
- PUVA,CALCIPOTRIOL.

Progressive Systemic Sclerosis

It is characterized by cutaneous and internal organ fibrosis. Raynaud's phenomenon is the earliest feature and may precede the onset of disease by:

- Is called CREST syndrome (Calcinosis, Raynaud's phenomenon, Esophageal dysfunction, Sclerodactyly and Telangiectasis).

American Rheumatism Association Criteria

Major

- Scleroderma proximal to the digits, affecting limbs, face, neck and trunk.

Minor

- Sclerodactyly.
- Digital pitted scarring.
- Bilateral basal pulmonary fibrosis.

One major criterion or two or more criteria suggest the diagnosis of systemic sclerosis.

Note: These criteria have 97% sensitivity and 98% specificity.

Cutaneous Manifestations

Hands and Feet

- *Early:* Raynaud's phenomenon.
- Painful ulceration at fingertips with pitted scars.
- **Late:** Sclerodactyly (induration of skin over the fingers) with tapering of fingers.
- Skin is tightly bound down.
- Leathery crepitations over joints and flexion contractures.
- Periungual telangiectasia.
- Bony resorption.

Face

- Periorbital edema is the early manifestation.
- Late manifestations include: Mask like facies, thinning of lips, microstomia, radial perioral furrowing, small sharp nose, telangiectasia and diffuse hyperpigmentation.

Trunk

- *Early:* Tense, stiff and waxy appearing skin that cannot be pinched and folded.
- *Late:* Impairment of respiratory movement of chest wall and of joint mobility.

  Other changes: **"Salt and pepper"** pigmentation, gangrene of fingers, mat like telangiectasia, leg ulcers and livido reticularis.

Organ involvement in PSS.

- Esophageal fibrosism, pulmonary interstitial fibrosis, myocardial fibrosis, small intestinal fibrosis, large intestinal fibrosis, renal involvement, skeletal muscle atrophy and thyroid fibrosis.

Investigation

- Skin biopsy.
- Nail fold capillary microscopy.
- ANA, Ab-SSA, SSB, Sm, nRNP **Scl-70 (specific for diffuse systemic sclerosis), anticentromere antibody (specific for CREST syndrome).**
- *Organ workup:* Urine analysis, barium swallow, esophageal manomerty, barium enema, chest X-ray and pulmonary function test.

Prognosis and cause of death

- Course of the disease is variable. Death occurs from intercurrent infection, hypertension and perforation of the gastrointestinal tract.

Other conditions where sclerodermoid changes are seen: (Pseudo scleroderma) Phenylketonuria, progeria, Rothmund-Thomson syndrome. Werner's syndrome, porphyria cutanea tarda, primary systemic amyloidosis, Hashimoto's disease, carcinoid syndrome, childhood diabetes mellitus and drugs (bleomycin, pentazocine, carbidopa and 5-hydroxytryptophan).

Treatment: Primarily directed towards complications. Pharmacological agents that used for systemic sclerosis can be grouped into various categories:

- Collagen modulators: D-penicillamine, relaxins and interferons.
- Vasoactive agents: Captopril, nifedipine and pentoxifylline.
- Immunosuppressive agents: Azathioprine, cyclophosphamide, cycloporine and methotrexate.

Dermatomyositis

Systemic, inflammatory disease involving primarily skin and muscles. Symmetric, proximal muscle weakness especially of the hips, thigh, and upper arm.

Proposed minimal set of hallmark cutaneous manifestations of DM for the purpose of defining amyopathic DM for future clinical studies.*

For this purpose, the hallmark cutaneous manifestations of DM are presumed to be present if the following conditions are met: presence of two major criteria or one major criterion and two minor criteria (biopsy of at least one skin lesion should show changes consistent with cutaneous DM).

Major Cutaneous Criteria

Heliotrope Rash

Macular violaceous erythema with or without associated scale of the eyelids or periorbital skin. Secondary or associated cutaneous findings, such as scale, pigmentary change, telangiectasia, or edema also can be present.

Gottron's Papules

Violaceous papules or small plaques overlying me dorsal or dorsal-lateral aspects of interphalangeal or metacarpophalangeal joints. When fully formed, these papules become slightly depressed at the center, which can assume a white, lacy appearance. Associated scale-hyperkeratosis, pigmentary change, or telangiectasia may be present.

Gottron's Sign

Macular violaceous erythema with or without associated scale-hyperkeratosis, pigmentary change, or telangiectasia involving extensor aspects of the knuckles, elbows, knees or medial malleoli.

Minor Cutaneous Criteria

Macular violaceous erythema (with or without associated scale-hyperkeratosis, pigmentary change, or telangiectasia) involving:

- Scalp → anterior hairline.
- Malar eminences of face, or forehead, or chin.
- V-area of neck or upper chest (open collar area; **V-sign**).
- Nape of die neck or posterior aspect of shoulders (**shawl sign**).
- Extensor surfaces of the arms or forearms.
- Linear streaking overlying extensor tendons on the dorsal aspects of the hands.
- Periungual areas.
- Lateral surface of thighs or hips (holster sign).
- Medial malleoli.

---

* These criteria were originally presented and discussed at the Third Annual Meeting of the Medical Dermatology Society in San Francisco on March 20th, 1997.

(Involvement of each above anatomic region qualifies as a single minor criterion).

Periungual nailfold telangiectasia or cuticular hemorrhage-infant with or without dystrophic cuticles.

Poikiloderma (concurrence of hyperpigmentation, hypopigmentation, telangiectasia, and superficial atrophy).

- **Mechanic's hand lesions.**
- Cutaneous calcinosis.
- Cutaneous ulcers.
- Pruritus.

Myositis-Specific Autoantibodies

Antisynthetase autoantibodies	
Jo-I	28 (16)
Other antisynthetases	5 (3)
SRP (Signal recognition particle)	5 (3)
Mi–2 (Antinuclear helicase and ATPase)	38 (21)

Myositis-Associated Autoantibodies

PM/Sel (Antiexosome complex)	10 (6)
Anticytoplasmic Ro/SS-A Ribonucleoproteins (RNPs)	
Ro60	8 (4)
Ro52	44 (24)
La/SS-B	6 (3)
UIRNP (Splicesome)	7 (4)

Treatment

- *Skin disease:* Topical steroids, hydroxychloroquine.
- *Muscle disease:* Systemic corticosteroids, azathioprine and methotrexate.

Overlap Syndrome

- The term overlap syndrome may be used when patients exhibit symptoms of more than one connective tissue disease.
- Such patients may meet diagnostic criteria for one disease but also have atypical manifestations or findings suggestive of second diagnosis.
- Systemic sclerosis combined with dermatomyositis is the most frequently seen overlap syndrome.

Mixed Connective Tissue Disease

- This entity was first described by Sharp and Colleagues.
- These patients, predominantly female, show features of SLE, systemic sclerosis, dermatomyositis and polymyositis.
- All patients have high titer of **antibody to U1 RNP (ribonucleoprotein).**
- Prominent clinical features include myositis, pulmonary hypertension, Raynaud's phenomenon, oesophageal hypomobility, swollen hands and sclerodactyly.

Sjögren's Syndrome (SS)

- Sjögren in 1933 described a triad of keratoconjunctivitis sicca, xerostomia and rheumatoid arthritis.
- Dry eyes and dry mouth occur in primary Sjögren's syndrome or if associated with other connective tissue disease then referred to as secondary Sjögren's syndrome.
- Most patients are aged 50 years or older and are women.
- Clinical feature include xerostomia, rhinitis sicca, vaginal dryness and dry eyes.
- Skin manifestations of SS include vasculitis, xerosis and annular erythema.
- Rheumatoid factor is usually positive.
- 80% of patients have anti Ro/SSA antibodies.
- Increased risk of developing lymphoreticular malignancies.
- No specific treatment available, only symptomatic management.

Lichen Sclerosus Atrophicus (LSA)

- It is chronic disease of the skin and mucous membrane of unknown origin predominantly affecting the females.

- Early lesions of LSA ivory white, polygonal, flat-topped papules or plaques with follicular plugs. The lesions may coalesce into large atrophic plaques.
- In women, involvement of the vulvar and perianal areas leads to the typical "figure of eight" or "hour glass" appearance.
- LSA of the penis in adults (Balanitis xerotica obliterans) presents with acquired phimosis or recurrent balanitis.
- LSA of vulva (Kraurosis vulvae) usually seen in postmenopausal women.
- LSA of the genitalia have increased risk for squamous cell carcinoma in women.
- **Treatment:** Medical–Topical steroids, topical testosterone, topical tretinoin. Surgical correction of adhesions may be required.

MULTIPLE CHOICE QUESTIONS

1. **Anti-histone antibodies are found in:**
   - A. DLE
   - B. SLE with pregnancy
   - C. Scleroderma
   - D. Drug induced LE
2. **Characteristic cutaneous involvement of dermatomyositis are all *except*:**
   - A. Gottron's papules
   - B. Heliotrope rash
   - C. Gottron's sign
   - D. Malar rash
3. **Anti-centromere antibody is found in:**
   - A. SLE
   - B. DLE
   - C. CREST
   - D. Childhood LE
4. **Anti-ds DNA antibodies in serum of a patient of SLE is associated with:**
   - A. High incidence of renal disease
   - B. Bad prognosis
   - C. CNS symptoms
   - D. Correlate directly with more extensive skin lesions
   - E. Both A and B
5. **Lupus-band test is immune deposits at dermo-epidermal junction of:**
   - A. Clinically normal, non-sun exposed skin
   - B. Clinically normal, sun exposed skin
   - C. Clinically involved, non-sun exposed skin
   - D. Clinically involved, sun exposed skin
6. **An early sign of scleroderma is:**
   - A. Raynaud's phenomenon
   - B. Sclenodactyly
   - C. Mask-like facies
   - D. Difficulty in swallowing
   - E. Round finger pad sign
7. **Civatte bodies (colloid bodies) are seen in:**
   - A. Lichen planus
   - B. SLE
   - C. Lichen Sclerosus et Atrophicus
   - D. All of the above
8. **ARA criteria for SLE includes all *except*:**
   - A. Serositis
   - B. Discoid rash
   - C. Oral ulcers
   - D. Photosensitivity
   - E. Lymphopenia < $1000/mm^3$
9. **The most common initial manifestation of SLE is:**
   - A. Pleuritic
   - B. Articular
   - C. Cutaneous
   - D. Fever
   - E. None of the above
10. **All factors contribute to etiology of scleroderma *except:***
    - A. Genetic
    - B. Vascular abnormalities
    - C. Excessive collagen deposition
    - D. T-helper cell function is increased
    - E. Metabolic
11. **All are side effects of d-Penicillamine *except*:**
    - A. Proteinuria
    - B. Thrombocytopenia
    - C. Pemphigus-like lesions
    - D. Pseudo-pseudo xanthoma elasticum
    - E. Psychosis

1 D 2 D 3 C 4 E 5 A 6 E 7 D 8 E 9 B 10 E 11 E

12. Poor prognostic factors for SLE—all *except*:
A. Male sex
B. Renal involvement
C. Anti-phospholipid syndrome
D. Thrombocytopenia
E. Asians and blacks
F. Haemolytic anaemia

13. Chloroquin is indicated in the treatment of:
A. Discoid LE
B. Lichen planus
C. Psoriasis
D. Dermatitis herpetiformis

14. Erosion of joints is seen in following *except*:
A. Psoriasis
B. Gout
C. Rheumatoid arthritis
D. SLE

15. Heliotrope erythema is a feature of:
A. SLE
B. Progressive systemic sclerosis
C. Morphea
D. Dermatomyositis

16. Calcinosis cutis is an indicator of good prognosis in:
A. Adult dermatomyositis
B. Childhood dermatomyositis
C. Scleroderma
D. SLE

17. Most sensitive test for diagnosing SLE is:
A. LE cell test
B. Direct immunofluorescence
C. Anti double stranded DNA antibody titre
D. Anti nuclear antibody titres

18. All are included in ARA criteria for SLE *except*:
A. Malar rash
B. Photosensitivity
C. Oral ulcers
D. Proteinuria exceeding 0.3g/day

19. Double stranded DNA antibody is best seen in:
A. SLE
B. Systemic sclerosis
C. Sq. cell carcinoma
D. Pemphigus

20. Scl 70 antibodies are associated with:
A. Dermatomyositis
B. CREST syndrome
C. Overlap syndrome
D. Diffuse scleroderma

21. Jo-1 antibody is associated with:
A. Dermatomyositis
B. Overlap syndrome
C. CREST
D. Morphea

22. LE Cell is a:
A. Lymphocyte B. Neutrophil
C. Keratinocyte D. Langerhan cell

23. Libman-sack endocarditis is a feature of:
A. Scleroderma
B. Pseudo-scleroderma
C. SLE
D. Dermatomyositis

24. All are causes of pseudo-scleroderma *except*:
A. PVC exposure
B. Rothmund-Thompson syndrome
C. Bleomycin
D. Diabetes
E. Raynaud's disease
F. Carcinoid syndrome

12 F 13 A 14 D 15 D 16 B 17 C 18 D 19 A 20 D 21 A 22 B
23 C 24 E

25. Drug induced SLE is characterized by all *except*:
- A. Males more commonly affected than female
- B. Anti-histone antibodies
- C. Older age group affected more frequently
- D. Renal + CNS involvement infrequent
- E. Anti-DNA antibodies absent

26. Death in SLE commonly occurs due to:
- A. Pulmonary embolism
- B. Renal failure
- C. Thrombocytopenia
- D. Endocarditis

27. Morphea is characterized by all *except*:
- A. Bound down skin
- B. Erythematous hue
- C. Asymptomatic
- D. Shiny surface

28. Which of the following is not true of chronic cutaneous LE?
- A. Discoid lesions are the hallmark
- B. Exposed areas, especially the face is involved
- C. Spontaneous remission occur in 25-40% of patients
- D. Hypertrophic lesions are seen in 2% of cases
- E. Many patients report flare ups during winter

29. All of the following cutaneous lesions can be found in SLE patients *except*:
- A. Mucous membrane lesions
- B. Scarring and non-scarring hair loss
- C. Livedo reticularis
- D. Kerato-conjunctivitis sicca
- E. Leg ulcers
- F. Necrobiosis lipodica

30. In SLE the most important pathologic change in connective tissue is:
- A. Fibrinoid change
- B. Oedema
- C. Proliferation of fibroblasts
- D. Inflammatory infiltrate

31. Anti RO and anti-La antibodies are found in all *except*:
- A. ANA negative SLE cases
- B. Neonatal LE
- C. SCLE
- D. DLE
- E. Complement deficient SLE

32. All of the following are used for treating DLE *except*:
- A. Topical steroids
- B. Chloroquine phosphate
- C. Etretinate
- D. Clofazimine
- E. Dapsone
- F. Vitamin C

33. UIRNP anti-bodies are seen in:
- A. Mixed connective tissue disorders
- B. Dermatomyositis
- C. Childhood LE
- D. Drug induced LE

34. Poor prognostic factors for SLE–all *except*:
- A. Male sex
- B. Renal involvement
- C. Anti-phospholipid syndrome
- D. Thrombocytopenia
- E. Asians and blacks
- F. Haemolytic anaemia
- G. Disorders of pigmentation

25 A 26 B 27 B 28 E 29 F 30 A 31 D 32 F 33 A 34 G

35. Calcinosis cutis is an indicator of good phognosis in:

A. Adult dermatomyositis
B. Childhood deumatomyositis
C. CREST syndrome
D. Progressive systemic sclerosis

36. En coup de sabre is:

A. Radiological appearance of tibia in congenital syphilis
B. Another name for collodian baluy
C. Morphoea of the fronto-parietal region
D. Another name for haulefuine foetus

37. 'White spot disease' commonly involves:

A. Face
B. Extremities
C. Vulva
D. Back

35 C 36 C 37 C

Chapter 6

Pigmentary Disorders

Vitiligo

Vitiligo is defined as a common, dermatological disorder characterized by well circumscribed, milky-white cutaneous macules **devoid of identifiable melanocytes.** It probably derived from the Latin word "vitium ("blemish"). Many ancient terms are applied to this condition–shwetakustha in the sacred Indian book, Atharva Veda (1400 BC), and sutra in Manusmriti (200 BC). In South India where the old Dravidian language of Tamil is spoken, the condition is known as *ven kushtam*—"white leprosy".

Pathogenesis

The white macules of vitiligo are the result of loss of melanocytes. The mechanism(s) by which the melanocytes are lost may be multiple but have not been identified unequivocally. Four hypotheses, not mutually exclusive, have been proposed to explain the causation of vitiligo:

- *Autoimmume:* Strengthened by the demonstation of specific autoantibodies to melanocyte cell surface antigens and the association of vitiligo with a variety of autoimmune disorders.
- *Autocytotoxic:* Also called as the self-destruction theroy, it proposes melanocyte destruction by intracellular retention of various precursor of melanin synthesis.
- *Neural:* Especially proposed to explain the segmental type of vitiligo.
- *Biochemical:* Accumulation of pteridines (6-biopterin and 7-biopterin) in the vitiliginous skin causes the depigmentation.
- *Intrinsic (genetic) theory:* An underlying genetic intrinsic factor predisposes some individuals to be more prone to develop vitiligo.

Clinical Features

- The diagnosis lesion of vitiligo is the typical vitiligo macule, which is of variable size, round/oval in shape, has a milky white color and scalloped margins.
- May appear at any age, however, the peak age at onset has been reported to be five to thirty years.
- Prevalence is the same in both sexes.
- The natural course of the disease is of progression, the lesions increasing both in number and size. In some cases there may be a rapid downhill course of vitiligo and this has been termed 'galloping vitiligo' or 'vitiligo fulminans'.
- Segmental vitiligo and vitiligo in children have a better prognosis.
- Mucous membrane involvement is also noted in vitiligo and is commoner, or rather, easily detectable in dark-skinned races.
- Leukotricha refers to depigmentation of the hair and may occur in some patients.

Classification of Vitiligo

Localized

- *Focal vitiligo*—This consists of one or more macules in one area but not clearly in a segmental or zosteriform distribution.
- *Segmental vitiligo*—Number of macules involving a unilateral segment of the body. The lesions stop abruptly and the midline of the affected segment.
- *Mucosal vitiligo*—Vitiligo affecting mucus membranes of the lips, oral cavity or the genitalia.

Generalized

- *Acrofacial vitiligo*—Lesions on the acral areas (hands and feet) and on the face, very often the perioral areas.
- *Vitiligo vulgaris*—Multiple macules of variable sizes over widely scattered areas often tending to bilateral symmery.
- *Lip-tip vitiligo*—Lesions affecting tips of the digits and the lips.
- *Mixed*—Any combination of vitiligo vulgaris and acrofacial vitiligo or of vitiligo vulgaris with segmental vitiligo.
- *Universal vitiligo*—This is the term used to describe complete or near complete depigmenation.

Special Signs in Vitiligo

- *Trichome vitiligo:* The trichome sign, also termed 'vitiligo gradata' describes a tan coloured zone (intermediate colour) between the normal skin and the depigmented macules. 'Quadrichrome vitiligo' implies the presence of fourth colour–dark brown–at the sites of perifollicular repigmentation.
- *Koebner's sign:* This phenomenon, a common feature of vitiligo, is defined as the development of lesions along the lines of specific trauma such as a cut, burn or abrasion. It may be a marker for disease activity.

Association of Vitiligo with Other Disease

- Vitiligo has been shown to be associated with autoimmune thyroid disease, Addison's disease, pernicious anaemia, diabetes mellitus and various dermatological disorder like alopecia areata, scleroderma, psoriasis and collagen vascular disorder. The Vogt Koyangi Harada syndrome is an apparently rare, multisystem disease characterized by vitiligo, poliosis, uveitis, dysacousia, and alopecia.

Treatment

Treatment of vitiligo can be broadly divided into medical and surgical modalities.

Medical Management

A. *Systemic*

- Psoralen (stimulates melanogenes in presence of ultraviolet radiation) UVA radiation (PUVA therapy).
- Corticosteroids (low dose twice weekly pulsed dosing of oral dexamethasone is safe and reasonably effective).
- Immunodulators (e.g. levamisole, cyclosporine, cyclophosphamide, azathioprine).
- Khellin (action similar to psoralens).
- Phenylalanine (+UVA).
- Antioxidants and nutritional supplements.

B. *Topical*

1. Topical PUVA.
2. Topical potent steroids.
3. Human placental extract.
4. Calcipotriol.
5. Topical pseudocatalase + calcium + UVB.
6. Cosmetic camouflage.
7. Dipigmenation with 20% monobenzyl ether of hydroquinone (for islands of residual repigmentation in extensive vitiligo).

Surgical Management

Indications

- Stable vitiligo (i.e. no new lesions for last two years).
- Refractory to medical management.

Modalities

- Punch grafting.
- Split skin thickness graft.
- Blister grafting.
- Melanocyte culture and transplantation.
- Tattooing.

Important Points

BEST treatment—Narrow band UVB therapy.
Localised disease (<20 %)—Topical therapy.
>20% - 50 %—Systemic therapy.
>50—Depigmentation.

Newer Topical Drug–Tacrolimus

Albinism

- Autosomal recessive inherited disorder.
- It is characterized reduced melanin synthasis in the melanocytes of the skin, hair and eyes, termed oculocytaneous albinism (OCA), and hypopigmentation primarily involving the retinal pigment epithelium of the eyes is fermed ocular albinism (OA).
- Due to genetic abnormalities of melanin synthesis associated with normal number and structure of melanocytes (differentiate it from vitiligo where melanocytes are reduced or absent).
- **Tyrosinase**-related OCA, the most common type of albinism is produced by loss of function of the melanocytic enzyme tyrosinase resulting from mutations of the tyrosinase gene.
- Affected individuals are born with white or blond hair and skin and blue eyes.

Piebaldism

- Piebaldism is an uncommon, autosomal dominant, congenital, stable leukoderma characterized by a white forelock and vitiligo-like amelanotic macules, usually containing a few normally pigmented or hyperpigmented macules.
- **Hyperpigmented macules within the amelanotic macules** and on normally pigmented skin are characteristic of piebaldism.

Pityriasis Alba

Pityriasis alba appears as superficial, pale pink to light brown macules with irregular, poorly circumscribed margins. It is round-to-oval in shape and can have slightly elevated borders. Initially the lesion starts as a subtle erythema, which progresses over weeks to produce the characteristic off-white macule with powdery scale.

Pityriasis alba is an eczematous dermatosis with hypomelanosis secondary to postinflammatory changes and the UV screening properties of the hyperkeratotic and parakeratotic epidermis.

Pityriasis alba lacks the complete depigmentation and distinct margins present in vitiligo. Mild topical corticosteroids with and without phototherapy, benzoic and salicylic acid in aquaphor, and 2% crude coaltar in petrolatum have been used with good results.

IMP: Face, Scaly, Dry skin.

Ash Leaf Macules

Ash leaf macules can be found in tuberous sclerosis, a neurocutaneous syndrome affecting multiple organs. **The classic triad is seizures, mental retardation, and adenoma sebaceum**. Cerebral hamartias (tubers) disrupt the brain structure and may cause seizure activity.

These hypopigmented macules occur in all ages of children. The size and shape of the lesions remain stable with age. They are about 1 to 3 cm in diameter, they can be located anywhere, and perifollicular pigment can appear within the lesion. On the posterior trunk, their long axes are in a transverse direction, whereas on the extremities they are cephalocaudal.

The **major cutaneous criteria for tuberous sclerosis are angiofibromas (adenoma sebaceum), fibrous plaques, and Koenen tumors**. Angiofibromas are often mistaken for acne lesions. These erythematous papules are in a malar distribution, occur after the second year of life, and are found in 80% to 90% of patients. Koenen tumors are periungual and subungual fibromas. Fibrous forehead plaques occur early in life and are believed to be angiofibromas.

Shagreen's patch is a connective tissue hamartoma that appears as an elevated pig skin like plaque on the lower back after the second year of life.

Waardenburg's Syndrome

WS (Waardenburg syndrome)—Hirschsprung disease or Shab-Waardenburg syndrome) is rare autosomal dominant disorder that is characterized by:

- Lateral displacement of the inner canthi and of lacrimal puncta.
- Prominence of the nasal root and of the medial eyebrows.
- Congenital deafness.
- Heterochromic irides.
- White forelock.
- Hypomelanotic macules.

Melasma (Chloasma)

- Melasma is a common acquired hypermelanois that occurs exclusively in sun-exposed areas; it is exacerbated by sun exposure, pregnancy, oral contraceptives, and certain anti-epilepsy drugs.
- Melasma presents in one of three usually symmetric facial patterns. The most common is a centrofacial pattern involving the cheeks, forehead, upper lip, nose and chin. Less common are the malar pattern, involving the cheeks and nose, and the mandibular pattern.
- Successful treatment of melasma involves the triad of sublocks, bleach and time.

Clinical points—(Female, pigmentation, cheeks).

Treatment

1. Inhibition of Tyrosinase activity or inhibit melanosome—Hydroquinone, azelaic acid, arbutin, kojic acid.
2. Desquamation of skin-tretinoin, glycolic acid, salicylic acid.
3. Anti-inflammatory-topical steroids.

KLIGMAN'S FORMULA—Hydroquinone, tretinoin, hydrocortisone.

Freckle (Ephelis)

It is an area of pale brown pigmentation usually less than 3 mm with poorly defined lateral margins

- Freckle appears as result of functionally overactive melanocytes with increase melanosomes (though, they are normal in number).
- They are seen only in fair skinned people.
- They are stimulated by ultraviolet radiation and fade away during winter.
- Histology reveals excess of melanin pigment in the basal layer.

Lentigo (Plural, Lentigines)

- Lentigo appears as a result of increased number of melanocytes in the basal layer.
- They does not show seasonal colour variations (not affected by ultraviolet radiation).
- Histology reveals linear increases of melanocytes in the basal layer.

Syndrome associated with lentigines

- **LEOPARD** syndrome—Lentigenes (multiple), ECG abnormalities, ocular abnormalities (hypertelorism), Pulmonary stenosis, Abnormalities of genitalia, Retardation of growth and Deafness (sensorineural).
- **NAME** syndrome—Nevi, Atrial myxoma, Myxoid neurofibromas and Ephelides.

- **LAMB** syndrome—Lentigines, Atrial myxoma, Mucocutaneous myxomas and Blue nevi.

Peutz-Jeghers Syndrome

- Peutz-Jeghers syndrome is an autosomal dominant disorder characterized by pigmented macules (lentigines) of **the buccal mucosa, lips, fingers and toes and by gastrointestinal polyps.**

DISORDERS OF HYPERPIGMENTATION

Pityriasis Versicolor

Pityriasis (tinea) versicolor is a superficial infection of the stratum corneum caused by the yeast Malassezia furfur (synonyms, Pityrosporum ovale, P. orbiculare). Young adults ages 15 to 35 are the most commonly affected age group, which is likely due to the higher lipid content of their skin. Cushing's syndrome, hyperhidrosis, immunosuppression, and malnutrition predispose to clinical infection.

Papulosquamous, follicular, and inverse patterns of pityriasis versicolor have been described. Papulosquamous lesions are the most common presentation and present initially as a reddish macule, which evolves into either a hypopigmented or a hyperpigmented superficial scaly plaque. The shape of the lesion may be nummular (coin shaped) or scalloped.

Sebaceous areas on the chest, back, abdomen, and proximal extremities are the most commonly involved sites.

Diagnosis is usually made by noting the charactersitic clinical appearance. Examination with a Wood's light may reveal a yellow-to-gold fluorescence. Skin scrapings may be examined under the microscope after the addition of 10% potassium hydroxide to confirm the diagnosis. Grapelike clusters of the yeast and short septate hyphae give a characteristic spaghetti and meatballs appearance on microscopy.

Eradication of pityriasis versicolor is difficult. Recurrence rates run as high as 60% to 80% within 2 years after treatment. Topical selenium sulfide 2.5% lotion is inexpensive, but prolonged application can cause local irritation.

Cafe Au Lait Macules

Ephelides and **cafe au lait** macules (CALM)—The latter are **most commonly associated with two disorders: Neurofibromatosis (NF) and McCune-Albright syndrome.**

CALM are flat, uniformly light brown in color, and can vary in size from 0.5 to 12 cm. 80% of adult patients with type I NF will have six or more CALM measuring 1.5 cm or greater in diameter. In comparison with NF, the **CALM in patients with McCune-Albright syndrome [polyostotic fibrous dysplasia with precocious puberty in females due to mosaicism for an activating mutation in a G protein (G_s?) gene]** are usually larger, more irregular in outline, and tend to respect the midline. CALM have also been associated with pulmonary stenosis (Watson syndrome), tuberous sclerosis, the LEOPARD syndrome, and ataxia telangiectasia, but a few such lesions can be found in normal individuals.

Acanthosis Nigricans

It appears as hyperpigmented, hyperkeratotic plaques with a velvetty texture. This **usually symmetric eruption affects the axillae, neck, groin, and breast folds most commonly** but may affect the antecubital fossae, popliteal fossae, perioral, and umbilical areas. Initially, it appears as a hyperpigmented macule that the patient refers to as a dirty area.

Benign acanthosis nigricans may present at birth. It is autosomal dominant with variable penetrance and has no relation to obesity. The most common form of acanthosis nigricans is that which is associated with obesity.

Malignant acanthosis nigricans is a cutaneous disorder that is a marker of an underlying malignancy. **Adenocarcinomas are the most commonly associated malignancies, with the stomach (60%) being the most frequent tumor location** followed by colon, ovary, pancreas, rectum and uterus. The tumor is present in 80% to 90% of patients at the time of the cutaneous manifestation.

Treatment of acanthosis nigricans is guided by its cause. Weight loss and treatment of underlying disorders can lead to a reversal of skin disease.

Postinflammatory Pigmentary Changes

Postinflammatory hyperpigmentation is an acquired increase in cutaneous melanin occurring after inflammation, whereas postinflammatory hypopigmentation is an acquired partial to total loss of melanin. Causes of postinflammatory pigmentary changes include infections, **allergic** reactions, papulosquamous disorders, medications, phototoxic eruptions, and physical agents.

DISORDERS OF KERATINIZATION

The ichthyosiform dermatoses is a heterogeneous group of disorders having scaling of the skin. *Ichthyosis* is derived from the Greek root *ichthy,* meaning fish.

MULTIPLE CHOICE QUESTIONS

1. **All of the following hyperpigmentation disorders are due to increased dermal melanocytes *except*:**
   A. Mongolian spot
   B. Naevus of ota
   C. Naevus of ITO
   D. Lentigines
2. **Vitiligo can be treated with:**
   A. Psoralens
   B. Topical steroids
   C. Systemic steroids
   D. All of the above
3. **The most common location of nevus anemicus is the:**
   A. Face
   B. Legs
   C. Trunk
   D. Neck
4. **Basal cell nevus syndrome is characterized by each of the following *except*:**
   A. Palmar pits
   B. Cerebral calcifications
   C. Bifid ribs
   D. Recessive inheritance
5. **Hydroquinone compounds cause depigmentation by their action on:**
   A. Melanocytes
   B. Tyrosinase
   C. DOPA
   D. Melanin
6. **Naevus anaemicus can be distinguished from naevus achromicus by the following tests:**
   A. Diascopy
   B. Intradermal injection of histamine
   C. Staining the skin sections for melanin
   D. All of the above
7. **Poikiloderma of civatte mainly involves:**
   A. Trunk
   B. Face and neck
   C. Extremities
   D. Scalp

1 D 2 D 3 C 4 D 5 B 6 D 7 B

Chapter 7

Disorders of Keratinization

Sl. No.	*Disorders*	*Onset*	*Type of scale*	*Sites*	*Histology*	*Other findings*	*Defect*
1.	Ichthyosis vulgaris	Childhood	Fine	Palms, soles, extensors	Diminished granular layer	Atopy, keratosis pilaris	Deficient **filaggrin**
2.	X-linked ichthyosis	Birth or infancy	Coarse, brown	Neck, face, trunk, flexors	Normal granular layer	Corneal opacities, cryptorchidism	Deficient **steroid sulfatase**
3.	Lamellar ichthyosis	Birth	Plate like, dark, erythroderma	Generalized with flexors, palms, soles	Increased granular lay, hyperkeratosis	Same as CIE	Unknown
4.	Epidermolytic hyperkeratosis	Birth	Erosions bullae coarse, verrucous later	Generalized, esp. flexors	Epidermolytic hyperkeratosis	Foul odor, pyogenic infections	Defect in keratins 1 and 10
5.	Congenital ichthyosiform erythroderma (CIE)	Birth	Fine, white, with erythroderma	Generalized with flexors, palms, soles	Increased granular layer, focal parakeratosis	Ectropion, nail dystrophy, poor growth, alopecia	Unknown
6.	Harlequin fetus	Birth	Massive thick plates	Generalized	Massive compact hyperkeratosis	Ectropion, eclabium, ear and limb deformities	Abnormal lamellar granules

Disorder	Inheritance	Incidence
Ichthyosis vulgaris	Autosomal dominant	1:250
X-linked ichthyosis	X-linked recessive	1:6,000
Epidermolytic hyperkeratosis	Autosomal dominant	
Congenital ichthyosiform erythroderma (CIE)	Autosomal recessive	
Lamellar ichthyosis	Autosomal recessive	
Harlequin fetus	Autosomal recessive	1:300,000 1:10001

Inheritance and incidence of the Major Congenital ichthyosis

COLLODION BABY

- A collodion baby is a newborn infant whose skin looks like a "baked apple", with a shiny, tough, membranous-like covering.
- It occurs in several types of ichthyosis like lamellar ichthyosis, Netherton's syndrome and Conradi's syndrome.
- Increased risk for infections and fluid and electrolyte imbalances due to cutaneous fissures and impaired barrier function of the skin.
- Treatment in a high humidity environment allows gradual sloughing of the collodion membrane.
- Manual debridement and keratolytics are not recommended.

Ichthyosiform Syndromes

Sjögren's-Larsson Syndrome

- An autosomal recessive disorder have metabolic defect, the deficiency of enzyme **fatty alcohol: nicotinamide-adenine dinucleotide oxidoreductase.**
- **Spastic diplegia, seizures, retinal glistening dots.**

Refsum's Syndrome

- Deficiency of enzyme phytanic acid oxidase with neurological and cutaneous clinical features.
- **Neurological changes include a cerebellar degenerative disorder (cerebellar ataxia), a progressive polyneuropathy, retinitis pigmentosa, and a sensory deafiness.** Rarely, cardiac abnormalities have been described.

KID Syndrome

- The acronym KID-Keratitis, Ichthyosis and Deafness describes the salient clinical features of this syndrome.

Netherton's Syndrome

- Ichthyosis linearis circumflexa, trichorrhexis invaginata (bamboo hair) and atopic dermatitis.

Acquired Ichthyosis

- Nutritional disorders.
- Metabolic disorders.
  Chronic renal failure results in hypervitaminosis A which produces rough, scaly skin.
- Drug therapy
  Niacin, triparanol, butyrophenones, dixyramine, and nafoxidine alter cholesterol synthesis. Cimetidine and the retinoids are antiandrogenic and reduce sebum secretion.
- Malignancies.

Treatment

- Topical emollients containing glycolic acid, lactic acid, urea, or glycerin may partially improve dryness and scaling. Topical tretinoin (Retin-A) is effective but poorly tolerated due to irritation.
- Oral retinoids, including isotretinoin, etretinate, and acetretin, are very effective, but relapses after treatment cessation are common.

Darier's Disease

- It is also known as keratosis follicularis and Darier-White disease, is an autosomally inherited disorder of keratinization that begins in the first or second decade of life.
- Histopathology shows changes of both premature keratinization and acantholysis.
- The primary lesions are flesh-colored papules that may coalesce into plaques and develop tan, scaly crusts.
- These keratotic papules are located in "seborrheic areas", such as the chest, back, ears, nasolabial folds, scalp and groin.
- Flat, wartlike papules may be seen on the dorsa of distal extremities, and 1-2 mm punctate

keratoses may be present on the palms and soles.

- Oral and rectal mucosal surfaces often demonstrate small, cobblestone-like papules.
- Nails demonstrate longitudinal ridging, as well as red and white longitudinal streaks. Distal nail edges show V-shaped notching and subungual thickening. Rarely, alopecia results from extensive scalp involvement.
- Histopath—*corps ronds, grains.*
- Topical and systemic retinoids are the drug of choice.
- Eczema, impetigo, fungal or viral infections, pemphigus vulgaris, pemphigus vegetans, or Darier's disease. The recurring, chronic nature of Hailey-Hailey disease, lack of oral and ocular involvement, and intertriginous predilection help to differentiate these conditions.

Clinical points (greasy, scales, seborhoeic areas, corps ronds, grains).

Palmoplantar Keratoderma (PPK)

Palmoplantar keratoderma is defined as thickening of palms and soles, which are genetically inherited or acquired.

Inherited PPK

- Inherited keratodermas may be a part of many genodermatoses but usually seen as an isolated feature.
- They can be inherited as an autosomal dominant or autosomal recessive trait. The important features of various inherited PPK are as follows:
  - **Thost-Unna (AD): Diffuse PPK:**
    * The **most common variety is the diffuse,** autosomal dominant palmoplantar keratoderma with livid red border *(tylosis).* Marked hyperhidrosis.
    * The thickening might be limited to the palmoplantar surfaces or extend on to the dorsal surfaces of palms and soles.
  - **Vorner type (AD):**
    * Diffuse PPK similar to Thost-Unna type. Histology shows **epidermolytic hyperkeratosis.**
  - **Vohwinkel's type (AD):**
    * Honey combed palmoplantar thickening with constriction bands and mutilation. **Star fish shaped keratosis on dorsa of hands and fingers.**
  - **Greither (AD):**
    * Diffuse PPK that is progressive. Extensor surfaces of hands, knees and elbows show psoriasiform plaque.
  - **Mal de Meleda (AR):**
    * Palmoplantar keratoderma in a glove like distribution. Erythema is prominent with hyperhidrosis and malodor.
  - **Papillon-Lefevre (AR):**
    * PPK associated with **periodontosis** and increased frequency of pyogenic infection.

Treatment

- Usually unsatisfactory.
- Keratolytics such as salicylic acid and urea can be used in higher concentrations.

Acquired Palmoplantar Keratodermas

- It is usually associated with some generalized skin conditions like psoriasis and pityriasis rubra pilaris.
- Some time many normal people have a few inconspicuous punctate keratoses on their palms and soles without any underlying systemic diseases.
- Keratoderma climactericum is seen in some women at about the time of menopause, most marked around the borders of the heels that causes painful fissuring and may interfere with walking.
- Paring and keratolytics generally help these patients. Hormone replacement may not help

but low dose of Acitretin will improve the condition.

Hailey-Hailey Disease

- Hailey-Hailey disease, also known as benign familial pemphigus, is an autosomal.
- Dominant condition characterized by localized patches of minute vesicles and erosions start in areas of friction, usually the neck, groin and axilla with itching, pain and foul odor.
- Histopath—**Dilapidated brick wall appearance.**
- Topical steroids are generally helpful in relieving burning and itching. Both *Staphylococcus aureus* and *Candida albicans* infections may exacerbate lesions, requiring treatment with appropriate antibacterial and antifungal agents. Recalcitrant cases have been treated with carbon dioxide laser, dermabrasion, topical cyclosporine, dapsone, vitamin E, PUVA, methotrexate, and thalidomide, with variable results.

Acanthosis Nigricans

Acanthosis nigricans is a nonspecific reaction pattern involving major body folds and mucocutaneous regions characterized by hyperpigmented, velvetty, soft, verrucous lesions in a symmetric fashion .

- Benign acanthosis nigricans involyes limited body areas and is less severe than malignant forms.
- Benign familial acanthosis nigricans, acanthosis nigricans associated with various syndromes, endocrine disease (especially insulin resistance diabetes mellitus), obesity (pseudoacanthosis nigricans) and drugs (Nicotinic acidic, fusidic acid, stillbestrol, oral contraceptives, triazinate).
- Malignant acanthosis nigricans is associated with extensive, widespread lesions and mucosal involvement.

Gastric carcinoma is the most commonly associated tumour.

MULTIPLE CHOICE QUESTIONS

1. Sex-linked ichthyosis vulgaris is associated with:
A. Transglutaminase deficiency
B. Steroids sulphatase deficiency
C. Elevated phospholipase c activity
D. Elevated adenylate cyclase activity

2. All of them cause acquired ichthyosis *except*:
A. Captopril
B. Nicotinic acid
C. Triparanol
D. Butyrophenone
E. Clofazimine

3. Following are characteristics of Darier's disease *except*:
A. Corps wounds in epidermis
B. Palms and soles may show minute pits
C. V-shaped notch over nails
D. Improves with UV radiation
E. Defect in tonofilament-desmosome complex

4. Granular layer is absent in which type of ichthyosis?
A. Ichthyosis vulgaris
B. X-linked ichthyosis
C. Harlequin foetus
D. Lamellar ichthyosis

5. Spot the wrong observation about ichthyosis:
A. Disorders of keratin formation
B. Ichthyosis vulgaris is not noticed until after 3 months of age
C. Sex-linked recessive variety starts soon after birth
D. Sex-linked recessive variety is seen in females only

6. Collodion baby is associated with:
A. Ichthyosis vulgaris
B. Lamellar ichthyosis
C. X-linked ichtyosis
D. Harlequin foetus

7. All are true of Harlequin foetus *except*:
A. Inherited as autosomal recessive
B. Ectropion, eclabium and small deformed ears
C. Hard fissured hyperkeratotic covering of the skin with fissuring
D. The infant is usually premature
E. Successful treatment with isotretinoin has been reported

8. All of the following are diagnostics criteria for neurofibromatosis *except*:
A. 6 or more café-au-lait macules of > 15 mm diameter in post-pubertal individuals
B. 2 more neurofibromas of any type or 1 plexiform neurofibroma
C. Axillary of inguinal freckling
D. 2 or more Lisch nodules
E. Phaechromocytoma

9. Mutilating palmoplantar keratoderma and peri-orificial involvement is seen in:
A. Melkarsson-Rosenthal syndrome
B. Papillion Lefevre syndrome
C. Proteus syndrome
D. Olmstead syndrome

1 B 2 A 3 D 4 A 5 D 6 B 7 E 8 E 9 D

10. A congenital syndrome consisting of macrodactyly, hemihypertrophy, exostoses, scoliosis, epidermalnevi, subcutaneous hamartomatous tumours and cerebri form thickening of the palms and soles is called:
A. Klippel-Trenaunay-Weber Syndrome
B. Proteus Syndrome
C. Gardner's Syndrome
D. Howel Evan's Syndrome

11. Which of the following is inherited as autosomal dominant?
A. Ichthyosis vulgaris
B. Lamellar ichthyosis
C. Epidermolytic hyperkeratosis
D. Congenital ichthyosiform erythroderma

12. Abnormal keratin profiles are found in all:
A. Ichthyosis vulgaris
B. Psoriasis
C. Darier's disease
D. Harlequin ichthyosis

13. All true of ichthyosis vulgaris *except*:
A. Autosomal dominant
B. Rarely present at birth
C. Improved with age
D. Scaling is worse on extension
E. Hair, nails teeth spared

14. Following is not true of bullous ichthyosiform erythroderma:
A. Autosomal dominant inheritance
B. Hyperkeratotic areas persist throughout life
C. Erythema and blistering increases as the child grows older
D. May present as a localized disorder only

15. Ichthyosis can be associated with all *except*:
A. Hypothyroidism
B. Hodgkin's disease
C. AIDS
D. Vitamin A deficiency
E. Mycosis fungoides
F. Hyperthyroidism

16. Crocodile skin of 'sauroderma' is seen in:
A. TEN
B. Psoriasis
C. Darier's disease
D. Ichthyosis vulgaris

17. The following are associated with ichthyosis vulgaris *except:*
A. Decreased sweating
B. Symptomatic treatment
C. Primarily involves flexor surfaces
D. Involves lipid abnormalities

18. All true of ichthyosis vulgaris *except*:
A. Autosomal dominant
B. Rarely present at birth
C. Improved with age
D. Scaling is worse on extension
E. Hair, nails, teeth spared

19. Kava, a psychoactive beverage with neuro-pharmacologic properties, may cause a dermopathy characterized by:
A. Vesiculobullous eruption
B. Atrophoderma
C. Lichenoid dermatitis
D. Ichthyosiform eruption

10 B 11 A 12 A 13 C 14 C 15 F 16 D 17 C 18 C 19 D

Chapter 8

Genetics in Dermatology

NEUROFIBROMATOSIS

Neurofibromatosis (NF) is one of the most common neurocutaneous conditions and consists of eight distinct forms of neurofibromatosis. The first two types are the most common and are autosomal dominant disorders with somewhat overlapping features: Neurofibromatosis type 1, also referred to as von Recklinghausen's disease, and the less common NF type 2.

Neurofibromatosis Type 1 (NF-1)

NF-1 is one of the most common autosomal dominant disorders in humans, with an occurrence of ~ 1 in 3000 persons. NF-1 accounts for 96% to 97% of all cases of NF and results from defects in the NF-1 gene on chromosome 17.

Etiology and Pathogenesis

The large gene for NF-1 is located on the long arm of chromosome 17 at 17 ql 1,2 and spans at least 300 kbp of DNA. Neurofibromin, the protein encoded by this gene, has several likely functions. This protein is essential for negative regulation of the rasproto-oncogene in the cell; therefore, it serves as a tumor suppressor.

Although NF-1 is inherited as an autosomal dominant disorder, 30% to 50% of cases are thought to result from spontaneous new mutations, most of which are paternal in origin. Somatic mosaicism for NF-1 has recently been identified. Some of the mosaic patients express disease in limited areas of the skin, a variant referred to as segmental NF.

Clinical Features and Presentation

In 1987, a panel convened at the National Institutes of Health and presented a consensus statement enumerating the clinical diagnostic criteria for NF-1 and NF-2.

For NF-1, the diagnostic criteria are met if two or more of the following features listed are present: (1) Six or more cafe-au-lait (CAL) macules greater than 5 mm in prepubertal patients and greater than 15 mm in postpubertal patients; (2) Two or more neurofibromas of any type, or one plexiform neurofibroma; (3) Axillary or inguinal freckling; (4) Optic nerve glioma; (5) Two or more Lisch nodules (iris harmatomas); (6) A distinctive osseus lesion such as sphenoid wing dysplasia or cortical thinning of long bones, with or without pseudoarthrosis; and (7) A first degree relative with NF-1 based on the preceding criteria.

CAL macules typically appear either at birth or during the first few years of an affected person's life. When CAL macules overlay the spine, this suggests the possibility of a plexiform neuroma and the potential of spinal dysraphism.

In patients with NF-1, the **most common benign tumor is a neurofibroma,** which may be either circumscribed (cutaneous or subcutaneous) or non-circumscribed (plexiform). For women, neurofibromas occur in almost 90% in the periareolar location; thus, breast examination is one of the best ways to detect subtle disease in an adult woman. Plexiform neurofibromas can wrap in and around vital structures and cause pronounced disfigurement, including compromised hearing. These are specific for NF-1. Optic nerve glioma is estimated to occur in 15% of patients with NF-1. Although these tumors usually develop by the time the patient is **10 years** old, symptoms of proptosis, decreased visual acuity, or precocious puberty (caused by pituitary compression) may not occur until years later. Treatment of optic nerve gliomas is often surgical and results in loss of vision; chemotherapeutic management is being investigated. Lisch nodules are iris hamartomas. Early development of Lisch nodules will be detectable with careful examination under a slit lamp by the **age of 6 years.** Distinctive osseus lesions of NF-1 include sphenoid wing dysplasia, which often results in pulsating exophthalmos or pseudoarthrosis of the tibia or fibula. This can predipose individuals to pathologic fractures and false joint formation. Only one long bone per patient is usually affected, and males are more commonly affected than females complications stenosis of the renal arteries, aqueduct stenosis, optic glioma, and learning disabilities; overt mental retardation is uncommon.

Malignant Risk

Patients with NF-1 have an estimated 3% to 15% lifetime risk of malignant disease—The two most common types of malignant tumors are neurofibrosarcoma and optic nerve gliomas. Other malignancies associated with NF-1 include malignant myeloid disorders, carcinoid, rhabdomyosarcoma, osteosarcoma, Wilm's tumor, ganglioneurofibroma, and medulloblastoma. Patients with NF-1 who also present with juvenile xanthogranulomas have been recently shown to have a greater statistical risk of developing chronic myelogenous leukemias.

Screening and Management

Diagnosis should be confirmed on the basis of outlined requirements, and should also include slit lamp examinations of all first-degree relatives of an index case, as well as a complete review of the condition, its inheritance pattern, and natural history.

Annual physical and ophthalmologic examinations during school years as well as audiology, speech, and language examinations before elementary school are recommended. Blood pressure should be checked once or twice a year. Growth abnormalities, scoliosis, and rapid enlargement or pain associated with neurofibromas should be monitored closely.

Neurofibromatosis Type 2 (NF-2)

NF-2, also known as central neurofibromatosis, accounts for about 3% of cases of NF and results from defects in the NF-2 gene on chromosome 27. Much less common than NF-1, the incidence of NF-2 is estimated at 1 in 50,000. Some evidence suggests that there are two subtypes of NF-2, a milder Gardner variant, and a more severe Whishart type.

Etiology and Pathogenesis

The gene for NF-2 is located on chromosome 22 at 22qll. In patients with NF-2, loss of heterozygosity for this region of chromosome 22 has been demonstrated in acoustic neuromas, neurofibromas and meningiomas.

Clinical Features and Presentation

The diagnostic criteria for NF-2 are either (1) Bilateral eighth nerve masses confirmed by CT or MRI or (2) A first-degree relative with NF-2 and either a unilateral eighth nerve mass or two of the following: neurofibroma, meningioma, glioma, schwannoma, or juvenile posterior subcapsular lenticular opacity.

Skin manifestations in NF-2 are less prominent than in NF-1. CAL tend to be fewer in number and show less distinct hyperpigmentation. Intertriginous freckling is not present. Neurofibromas, especially the plexiform variant, are the least common cutaneous finding in NF-2.

One characteristic skin finding includes cutaneous and subcutaneous schwannomas, the most common of the various tumors seen in NF-2. Schwannomas typically present as superficial, discrete, slightly raised papules in which the surface is rough, often pigmented, and covered by excess hair.

Tuberous Sclerosis Complex

Tuberous sclerosis complex (TSC) is the second most common neurocutaneous disorder. The transmission is autosomat dominant; however, ~65% to 85% of cases arise from spontaneous mutations. In 1908, Vogt described the classic triad of adenoma sebaceum, seizures, and mental retardation, but less than a third of patients display all of these features.

Etiology and Pathogenesis

Tuberous sclerosis is a disorder of cellular differentiation and proliferation. Two TSC genes have been identified; one is on chromosome 9q34 (TSC1) and the other is on chromosome 16pl3 (TSC2).

Clinical Features and Presentation

Cutaneous findings include hypomelanotic macules, facial angiofibromata, ungual fibromas and the shagreen patch. Hypomelanotic macules are seen in at least 90% of affected patients, but these lesions are not specific for tuberous sclerosis because one or two often occur in the general population.

The **earliest** detectible abnormalities in TS are **hypopigmented macules and rhabdomyomas,** both of which are often present at birth. Facial angio fibromata are found in 75% of all patients with tuberous sclerosis. Ungual fibromas are fleshy lesions that occur beneath the nails. They occur in only 25% of affected persons, arise in early adulthood, and are fairly specific for tuberous sclerosis. A shagreen patch is a cluster of connective tissue hamartoma that appears as an irregularly shaped plaque with a green to red hue, and is commonly found on the patient's back or flank.

Central nervous system lesions of tuberous sclerosis include cortical hamartomas (tubers), focal cortical dysplasia, subependymal nodule, subependymal giant cell astrocytoma, and retinal phakoma (astrocytomas). Renal involvement exists in upto 80% of patients and may lead to significant morbidity and mortality. One study cited renal disease as the leading cause of death in adults with tuberous sclerosis. Angiomyolipomas are by far the most frequent renal lesion, and the risk of hemorrhagic complications appears to be related.

Screening and Management

Prenatal diagnosis is difficult because genetic transmission can be from one of two chromosomes and the majority of cases are actually new mutations. Family members should undergo a physical examination with Wood's lamp to accentuate Ash-Leaf spots and dilated funduscopy to delineate retinal phakomas. For inherited cases, genetic counselling of parents is important because ~ 50% of offspring will be afflicted.

Von Hippel-Lindau Disease (VHL)

VHL also referred to as CNS angiomatosis - retinal angiomatiosis in 1904. Cutaneous findings are portwine stains and café-au-lait macules. Dermal capillary malformation has predilection for the head and neck. Other manifestations are vascular malformations in the cerebellum and brainstem. Retina is also commonly affected. There may be cystic neoplasms or angiomatous lesions in the kidneys, liver and pancreas.

Sturge-Weber Syndrome

- Sturge-Weber syndrome (SWS) is defined as facial portwine stain in association with ipsilateral plial (i.e. leptomeningeal) vascular anomalies (with one or more symptoms; epilepsy early in life, hemiparesis or hemiplegia, gyriform intracranial calcifications and cerebral atrophy) and inconstant ipsilateral choroidal vascular lesions with glaucoma.
- Xeroderma pigmentosum (Pigmented dry skin).
- It is an autosomal recessive disorder characterized by photosensitivity, pigmentary changes, premature skin aging, neoplasia and abnormal DNA repair.
- Eight different subtypes—complementation groups A to G and XP variants.
- Main defect is in the DNA excision repair process (this is a process whereby damaged DNA is replaced with new DNA).
- Earliest symptoms of dryness and freckling appear between six months and three years of age.
- Next is the poikilodermatous stage characterized with atrophy and telangiectasia superadded to the existing freckles and hyperpigmentation.
- Pre-malignant lesions like actinic keratosis and keratoacanthomas may occur in most cases.
- Patients with XP under 20 years of age have a greater than 1000 fold increased risk of cutaneous basal cell or squamous cell carcinoma or melanoma. The median age of onset of nonmelanoma skin cancer reported in patients with XP was 8 years.

Incontinentia Pigmenti

- Incontinentia pigmenti is an uncommon genodermatosis of the developing neuroectoderm in which vesicular, verrucous and pigmented lesions are associated with developmental defects of eye, skeletal system and central nervous system.
- Incontinentia pigmenti is a complex hereditary syndrome that principally affects female infants. It is inherited as an X-linked dominant disorder.

MULTIPLE CHOICE QUESTIONS

1. Which of the following is true for Ash-Leaf macules?
- **A.** Ovate or lanceolate hypopigmented macules
- **B.** They have dermatomes distribution
- **C.** They are the earliest cutaneous markers of EPILOIA
- **D.** The lesion vary from 1 to100
- **E.** All of the above
- **F.** A and C are correct

2. Crowe's sign is:
- **A.** 6 or more café-au-lait macules
- **B.** Radiologic sign showing bony lesion in NF-1
- **C.** Diffuse freckling of axillae and other body fold
- **D.** Another name for plexiform neurofibroma

3. All true of Sturge-Weber syndrome *except*:
- **A.** Inherited as autosomal dominant with variable penetrance
- **B.** Fascial port-wine stain
- **C.** Homolateral leptomeningeal andiomatosis
- **D.** Portwine stains are present on the extremities or trunk in addition to face in 40% of cases
- **E.** Portwine stain may be bilateral

4. Werner's syndrome presents with the following dermatological features *except*:
- **A.** Premature graying of hair
- **B.** Hirsutism
- **C.** Atrophy of skin
- **D.** Atrophy of subcutaneous tissue

5. 'Coast of Maine' appearance is seen in:
- **A.** Mc Cure Albrights
- **B.** Neurofibromatosis
- **C.** Tuberous sclerosis
- **D.** Piebaldism

6. Xeroderma pigmentosum is produced as a result of defect in:
- **A.** DNA polymerase III
- **B.** DNA polymerase I
- **C.** DNA exonuclease
- **D.** DNA ligase

7. All are features of tuberous sclerosis *except*:
- **A.** Shagreen patch
- **B.** Mental retardation
- **C.** Ash leaf macule
- **D.** Lisch nodule on iris

8. Sex-linked ichthyosis vulgaris is associated with:
- **A.** Transglutaminase deficiency
- **B.** Steroids sulphatase deficiency
- **C.** Elevated phospholipase activity
- **D.** Elevated adenylate cyclase activity
- **E.** Defect in tonofilament—desmosome complex

1 F 2 C 3 A 4 B 5 A 6 D 7 D 8 B

9. All true of Harlequin foetus *except*:
A. Inherited as autosomal recessive
B. Ectropion, eclabium and small deformed ears
C. Hard fissured hyperkeratotic covering of the skin with fissuring
D. The infant is usually premature
E. Successful treatment with isotretinoin has been reported

10. Common skin lesions seen in tuberous sclerosis *except*:
A. Ash-Leaf macules
B. Facial angiofibromas
C. Shagreen patch
D. Koener's tumors
E. Axillary frecking

11. Incontinentia pigmenti is characterized by all *except*:
A. Vesiculobullous lesions
B. Hyperpigmentation
C. Telangiectases
D. Verrucous lesions
E. Hypopigmentation

12. Malignancies which can be associated with NF-1 are all *except*:
A. Neuro fibrosarcoma
B. Phaecheromocytoma
C. Wilm's tumor
D. Rhabdomyosarcoma
E. Leukemia
F. Osteosarcoma

13. Tuberous sclerosis is linked genetically to:
A. Chromosomes 17 and 22
B. Chromosomes 9 and 16
C. Chromosomes 11 and 22
D. Chromosome 12

14. Ataxia-telangiectasia—all true *except*:
A. Autosomal dominant inheritance
B. Defective gene on region 22 and 23 of chromosome 11q
C. Progressive cerebellar ataxia is the earliest clinical manifestation
D. Muco-cutaneous telangiectasias
E. Severe respiratory infections and lymphoreticular malignancies are the two most common causes of death

15. Vohwinkel's syndrome is characterized by the following *except*:
A. Hyperkeratosis of palms and soles
B. Hyperhidrosis
C. Syringobulbia
D. Hypogonadism

16. Conradi-Hunter syndrome is characterized by following *except*:
A. Mild to moderate growth deficiency
B. Low nasal bridge
C. Scoliolosis
D. Alopecia is common

17. Vogt-Koyanagi-Harada syndrome comprises:
A. Involvement of brain and meninges
B. Bilateral uveities, labyrinthitis and deafness
C. Poliosis, leucoderma, alopecia
D. All of the above
E. None of the above

18. Wardenberg's syndrome is comprised all *except:*
A. Heterochromia of iris
B. Saddle shaped nose
C. Lateral displacement of inner canthi
D. Deafness
E. Poliosis

9 D 10 E 11 B 12 B 13 B 14 A 15 C 16 D 17 D 18 A

19. Leukoderma in tuberous sclerosis is due to:

A. Impaired melanosome transfer
B. Decreased tyrosin activity
C. Decreased number of melanocytes
D. None of the above

20. All are true of Hypomelanosis of Ito *except*:

A. Unilateral or bilateral streaks of hypopigmentation
B. Lesions usually appears by 1 year of age
C. An initial increase in extent of involvement followed by gradual repigmentation
D. Dermal melanophages
E. Streaks of hypopigmented hairs

21. Leopard syndrome is also known as:

A. Generalized lentigenosis
B. Multiple lentigenes syndrome
C. Eruptive lentigenosis
D. Zostriform lentigenosis
E. Centrofacial lentigenosis

22. Cafe-au-lait macules (CALM) are associated with all *except*:

A. Neurofibromatosis
B. McCune Albright syndrome
C. Fanconi's syndrome
D. Acropigmentation of kitamura

23. Naevus depigmentosus all true *except*:

A. Usually presents in second year of life
B. Lesions may be multiple
C. Lesions may be in dermatomal or whorled pattern
D. Defect in transfer of melanosomes to keratinocytes has been postulated

24. The gene for NF-1 is located on:

A. Chromosome 14
B. Chromosome 12
C. Chromosome 9
D. Chromosome 17

25. Diagnostic criteria for NF-2 include all *except*:

A. Bilateral acoustic neuromas
B. First degree relative with NF-2
C. Unilateral VII nerve mass
D. Axillary freckling

26. All true of Lisch nodules *except*:

A. Melanocytic hamartomas of the iris
B. When multiple, they are pathognomonic of NF-1
C. Occur in >90% of patients of NF-1 by second decade of life
D. Best seen by naked eye

27. Most common CNS tumor occurring in NF-1:

A. Astrocytoma
B. Schwannomas
C. Optic glioma
D. Oligo-dendritoma

28. Characteristic ocular sign of NF-2:

A. Optic glioma
B. Lisch nodules
C. Posterior subcapsular cataracts
D. Heterochromia of the iris

29. Earliest skin sign of tuberous sclerosis:

A. Café-au-lait macules
B. Ash-Leaf macules
C. Crowe's sign
D. Ichthyosis

30. Incontinentia pigmenti is characterized by all *except*:

A. Vesiculobullous lesions
B. Hyperpigmentation
C. Telangiectasia
D. Verrucous lesions
E. Hypopigmentation

---

19 A 20 D 21 B 22 D 23 A 24 D 25 D 26 D 27 C 28 C 29 B
30 C

31. Plain X-ray skull taken in later childhood in patients of tuberous sclerosis reveals:
A. Punched out lesions of the skull
B. Bilateral areas of calcification in the brain
C. Cystic areas in the brain
D. Cortical tubers

32. Which cardiac abnormality is characteristic of tuberous sclerosis?
A. Atrial septal defect
B. Congenital rhabdomyoma
C. Boot-shaped heart
D. Ventricular septal defect

33. Fundoscopic examination in tuberous sclerosis reveals:
A. Retinal haemorrhage
B. Calcification
C. Phacoma
D. Optic glioma

34. Typical appearance seen on X-ray skull in later childhood of patients with Sturge-Weber syndrome is:
A. Periventricular calcification
B. Tram-track calcification
C. Vascular abnormalities
D. Intracranial space occupying lesion

35. All true of ocular complication in Sturge-Weber syndrome:
A. Occur in 30-60% cases
B. Capillary malformations of conjunctiva, iris and choroid
C. Glaucoma
D. Megalocornea
E. Optic glioma is found in 20% cases

36. Treatment of choice for facial portwine stain:
A. Argon LASER
B. Tunable pulsed dye laser
C. Nd-yag LASER
D. Ruby LASER

37. Von-Hippel-Lindau disease—all true *except*:
A. Facial or occipito-cervical portwine stain
B. Autosomal recessive
C. Bilateral retinal angiomatosis
D. Renal cell carcinoma
E. Cerebellar hemangioblastoma

38. Ataxia-telangiectasia—all true *except*:
A. Autosomal dominant inheritance
B. Defective gene on regions 22 and 23 of chromosome 11q
C. Progressive cerebellar ataxia is the earliest clinical manifestation
D. Mucocutaneous telangiectasias
E. Severe respiratory infections and lymphoreticular malignancies are the two most common causes of death

39. The following naevi contains the naevus cells:
A. Naevus of ota
B. Epidermal naevus
C. Lymphangioma circumscriptum
D. Naevus acromicus

40. Surgical excision is necessary in:
A. Halo naevus
B. Giant pigmented naevus
C. Muscular pigmented naevus
D. Naevus of ota

41. Adenoma sebaceum is commonly mistaken for:
A. Boils
B. Acne
C. Psoriasis
D. Lymphoma

31 B **32** B **33** C **34** B **35** E **36** B **37** B **38** A **39** A **40** B **41** B

42. Papillion Lefevre syndrome is characterized by the following *except*:
A. Calcification of falx cerebi and tentorium cerebelli
B. Periodontosis
C. Vitiligo
D. Palmoplantar hyperkeratosis

43. Proteus syndrome is characterized by the following *except:*
A. Epidermal naevi
B. Macrodactyly
C. Thick tongue
D. Subcutaneous tumours

44. Skin biopsy is most helpful in the diagnosis of incontinentia pigmenti during:
A. Vesicular stage (stage 1)
B. Verrucous stage (stage 2)
C. Pigmentary stage (stage 3)
D. Atrophic stage (stage 4)

45. In infants and young children, the earliest sign of xeroderma pigmentosum is:
A. Unusually severe sun sensitivity with blistering
B. Development of premalignant actinic keratoses
C. Growth retardation
D. Sensory neural hearing loss

46. A laboratory test may be used to diagnose Wegener's granulomatosis is:
A. Anticentromere antibody
B. Antineutrophil chemotaxis antibody
C. Rapid plasma reagin
D. Anti-double stranded DNA

47. Basic defect in xeroderma pigmentosum is:
A. A lack of normal capacity to repair ultraviolet radiation damage to DNA
B. The defective DNA synthesis
C. The defective RNA synthesis
D. Lack of normal capacity to repair ultraviolet radiation damage to RNA

48. The following skin diseases display autosomal dominant inheritance:
A. Hereditary haemorrhagic telangiectasia
B. Tuberous sclerosis
C. Phenyiketonuria
D. Xeroderma pigmentosum
E. Neurofibromatosis

49. Ocular hallmark of pseudoxanthoma elasticum is:
A. Retinal hemorrhage
B. Iritis
C. Angoid streak
D. Keratitis

50. Which of the following mode of inheritance is associated with Fabry disease?
A. Autosomal dominant inheritance
B. Autosomal recessive inheritance
C. Sex-linked inheritance
D. No known heritable tendency

51. Beaded margins of eyelids is a characteristic feature of:
A. Granuloma annulare
B. Leprosy
C. Erythema annulare centrifugum
D. Lipoid proteiniosis

42 C 43 C 44 A 45 A 46 B 47 A 48 A,B,E 49 C 50 C 51 D

Chapter 9

Eczema and Dermatitis

Eczema is an inflammatory skin reaction characterized histologically by spongiosis with varying degrees of acanthosis, and a superficial perivascular lymphohistiocytic infiltrate. The clinical features of eczema may include itching, redness, scaling and clustered papulovesicles. Cutaneous inflammation is called as dermatitis and the terms dermatitis and eczema are now-a-days generally regarded as synonyms.

Classification

A. **Exogenous eczemas**

1. Irritant contact dermatitis.
2. Allergic contact dermatitis.
3. Photo allergic contact dermatitis.
4. Eczematous polymorphic light eruption.
5. Infective dermatitis.
6. Dermatophytide.
7. Post-traumatic eczema.

B. **Endogenous eczemas**

1. Atopic dermatitis.
2. Seborrheic dermatitis.
3. Asteatotic eczema.
4. Discoid eczema.
5. Exudative discoid and lichenoid dermatitis.
6. Chronic scaly superfical dermatitis.
7. Pityriasis alba.
8. Hand eczema.
9. Gravitational eczema.
10. Juvenile plantar dermatosis.
11. Metabolic eczema or eczema associated with systemic disease.
12. Eczematous drug eruptions.

A. *Exogenous eczemas:* The common types are:

1. *Irritant contact dermatitis:* This is an inflammatory reaction of the skin to an external agent or agents. Although inflammatory and immunological mediators may be activated, no memory T-cell function or antigen-specific immunoglobulins are involved.

Common irritants are detergents, soaps, solvents and abrasives, alkalies, acids, oxidizing agents, reducing agents, animals enzymes and secretions and desiccant powders, dust and soil.

The common occupations are hairdressing, medical, dental, agriculture, catering, printing and painting, mechanical engineering, fishing and construction etc.

Clinical features: Varied clinical presentations may be seen ranging from dry lichenified erythematous lesions of chronic dermatitis to erythematous, exudative crusted, papulovesiculobullous lesions of acute dermatitis depending on the duration of contact, irritant potential and concentration of the irritant.

2. *Contact allergic dermatitis*: Dermatitis developing after weeks to years of

repeated contact with allergen is quite common. This is mediated through delayed or cell mediated type of immunity and occur due to many dyes and their intermediates, oils, resins, coaltar derivatives, chemicals used for fabrics, rubbers, cosmetics, insecticides, oils and resins of woods and plants as well as products of bacteria, fungi and parasites.

Clinical features: Erythema, swelling, papules and vesicles and on constant scratching lichenification develops. With specific allergens erythema multiforme like, purpuric reactions, lichenoid, papular eruptions, pigmentation and granulomatous reactions may develop.

B. *Endogenous eczemas:* The common ones are:

1. *Atopic dermatitis*: It is an itchy, chronic or chronically relapsing inflammatory skin disease. Onset is between 2 and 6 months in the majority of cases. With features of itching, macular erythema papules and papulovesicles eczematous areas with crusting, lichenification and excoriation, dryness of skin and secondary infection. Distribution varies with age:
   a. *Infantile phase:* Lesions start on face and may occur on any area but usually spare napkin area. When the child starts crawling extensor surfaces are more involved.
   b. *Childhood phase:* From 18-24 months onwards characteristic sites like elbow and knee flexors, sides of neck, wrists and ankles are involved.
   c. *Adult phase:* It involves mainly flexors and hand. Associated features of atopic dermatitis could be asthma, hay fever, dry skin, alopecia areata, urticaria, food allergy and drug sensitivity. It is a chronic disorder which usually improves with age and most of the people show remission by the age of puberty.
2. *Seborrheic dermatitis:* It is a dematitis of predominantly seborrheic areas involving scalp, eyebrows, nasolabial folds, chin, presternal and interscapular regions, axillae and groins. Lesions are erythematous, scaly and diffuse plaques or patches with waxy, yellowish scales. The most common etiological agent implicated is an yeast, Malassezia ovale.
3. *Pityriasis alba:* It is a nonspecific superficial dermatitis of unknown origin and has been regarded as a manifestation of atopic dermatitis.

   Rounded oral or irregular phaques which are red, pink or skin coloured are seen over face, mainly around mouth, chin and cheek. On healing they leave hypo pigments scaly patches.
4. *Hand eczema*: The term hand eczema implies that the dermatitis largerly confined to the hands with only minor involvement of other areas.

   The common morphological variants are pompholyx, recurrent focal palmar peeling, fingertip eczema and patchy vesiculosquamous type. Pompholyx is more common in 10-40 years age group and presents with crops of clear vesicles. Itching is usually severe and resolves in 2-3 weeks.

   Recurrent focal palmar pending was initially known as keratolysis exfoliative. During summer months small area of superficial white desquamation develop on the sides of the fingers and on the palms or on the feet.

   Fingertip eczema involves mainly thumb and forefingers of dominant hand and presents as dry, cracked or painful fissuring of the skin. It is usually worse in winter and improves in holidays.

   Patchy vesiculosquamous type presents as asymmetrical patchy, irregular vesicles and scaly lesions on both hands.

Histopathology of various stages of eczema. Spongiosis, acanthosis, vascular dilation of papillary dermis and lymphohistocytic dermal infiltrate are almost always seen.

1. *Acute stage*: Spongiosis and vesicle formation predominate.
2. *Subacute stage*: Spongiosis and vesiculation diminish and acanthosis increases. Parakeratosis is seen. In later stages rete ridges becomes elongated and broadened.
3. *Chronic stage:* Hyperkeratosis coexists with parakeratosis, cells no longer invade epidermis and dermal changes become prominent.

Diagnosis 1: On the basis of history, clinical features and patch testing with the standard battery of allergens which is now commercially available.

Treatment of Eczemas

A. *General measures*

1. Reassurance and counselling of patient and parents regarding the trigger factor, treatment options, benefits and risks.
2. Protection from different chemicals and allergens with the help of wet mopping of floor, wearing of full sleeve clothes, gloves etc.
3. To avoid excessive drying or wetting of skin with regular bathing and frequent topical application of emollients.

B. *Specific measures*

1. **Oral therapy:**

   Antibiotics—If the lesion shows vesiculation and apparent infection, patient may be given antibiotics which cover mainly staphylococcus and streptococcus like Erythromycin and Cloxacillin.

   Antihistamines—H_1 receptor antagonists like promethazine etc can be given in liberal amount to decrease itching and also for sedation.

   Others: Low dose cyclosporin, evening primrose oil, oral corticosteroid, Chinese herbal medicines, sodium cromoglycate, azathioprine, interferon gamma etc. has been tried with variable success.

2. **Topical therapy:** *Topical steroids*—They are the most commonly used agents. For acute eczemas super potent steroids can be used and after controlling the disease moderately potent steroids can be started. Less potent steroid is needed for infants and on areas such as eyelids, face, genitalia and axillae.

   For chronic cases steroids can be used under occlusion but it can cause infection, atrophy and other side effects.

   Ichthammol and tar: Preparations containing ichthammol and tar can be helpful as maintenance treatment in patients with lichenification.

   Antifungals: For seborrheic dermatitis topical selenium sulphide in shampoo base or topical terbinafine or ketoconazole can be used effectively to decrease M. Ovale load.

C. *Other measures:* UV radiation—Physiotherapy with UVB or UVA or combination of the two are helpful in atopic dermatitis, principles of local therapy of contact dermatitis.

ATOPIC DERMATITIS (II)

- The term 'Atopy' meaning "out-of-place-ness" or different was coined by **Coca** in 1923.
- It refers to predisposition to develop asthma, allergic rhinitis and atopic dermatitis.
- Atopic patients have:
  - Blood and tissue eosinophilia.
  - Increased IgE responses.
  - Increased transepidermal water loss.
  - Increased sensitivity to pruritic stimuli.
  - Immune system dysfunction associated with decreased cell mediated immunity.

Therapeutic agent	*Acute*	*Subacute*	*Chronic*	*Prophylactic*
Wet dressings	++	±	–	–
Creams, lotions	++	+	±	–
Pastes	–	+	++	–
Emollients	±	±	+	+
Corticosteroids, local	±	++	++	–
Immunosuppressants, local	±	+	++	–
Tar, ichthammol, etc.	–	±	++	–
Polythene occlusion	–	+	++	±
Paste bandage occlusion	–	+	++	–
Intralesional steroids	–	±	++	–

- Exact cause is not known but 70% patients have a family history of at least one of the three atopic disorders.
- Psychological, climatic and immunologic factors are also responsible.

Rajka: These are generally used for clinical research. Major criteria include:

- Pruritus.
- Flexural lichenification.
- Chronically relapsing course.
- A personal or family history of atopy.

There are 23 minor criteria, the most relevant of which are:

- Xerosis.
- Ichthyosis.
- Immediate skin test reactivity.
- Elevated serum IgE.
- Early age of onset.
- Tendency for developing cutaneous infections.
- Tendency for developing non-specific hand or foot dermatitis.
- Dennie-Morgan infraorbital fold.
- Keratoconus.
- Anterior subcapsular cataracts.
- Orbital darkening.
- Facial pallor/erythema.
- Pityriasis alba.
- Itch when sweating.
- Intolerance to wool and lipid solvents.
- Perifollicular accentuation.
- Food intolerance.
- The influence of emotional factors.
- White dermographism/delayed blanch.

To fulfil the criteria, the patients must have three or more of the major and three or more of the minor criteria. Additional features identified in patients are scaling of the scalp and infra-auricular fissures.

The presence of atopic syndrome can be confirmed by serum testing (i.e. radioallergosorbent test or RAST) or by intracutaneous challenge, looking for allergen-specific IgE antibodies to:

- House dust.
- House dust mite.
- Pollen (tree/grass/weed).
- Animal dander (cat/dog).
- Moulds.

If atopy is not confirmed (in upto 10% of the patients with the clinical diagnosis according to the criteria of Hanifin and Rajka) by this test (or by the use of a skin-prick test) the test should be repeated at a later point in time. This is especially applicable in small children.

- Kaposi's varicelliform eruption is a dramatic and uncommon complication of atopic dermatitis. It involves widespread infection of dermatitis skin with umblicated vesicles due to herpes simplex (eczema herpeticum), vaccinia (eczema vaccinatum) or coxsackie A16 viruses (eczema coxsackium).
- Factors provoking or exacerbating atopic dermatitis are:
  - – Excessive washing without proper lubrication of skin.

- Wool, synthetic fabrics, poorly fitting clothes, mineral oils, solvents, sand and excessive perspiration.
- Airborne particles like smoke, animal dander moulds, house dust mites.
- Secondary infections due to *Staphylococcus aureus* or *Pityrosporum orbiculare*.
- Foods like milk, eggs, nuts, soy, wheat, seafood have been incriminated but role remains controversial.

• Atopic dermatitis may begin at any age although 60% develop it within the first year of life and 90% by fifth year.

• Four phases are commonly recognized.

1. **Infantile Phase** (2 months–2 years)
   • Characterized by intense itching, erythema, papules, vesicles, oozing and crusting.
   • Eruptions seen typically on cheeks, forehead, scalp, less on the trunk and extremities diaper area—usually spared.
   • Dermatitis clears in 50% of patients by 3 years of age.
2. **Childhood phase** (3-11 years)
   • More chromic, lichenified lesions present as circumscribed scaly patches.
   • Classic areas include the wrists, ankles, back of thighs, buttocks, antecubital and popliteal fossae.
   • 75% of patients clear by age of 6 years.
3. **Adolescent young adult phase** (12-20 years)
   • Thick, dry, lichenified, plaques are seen on the face, neck, upper arms, back and flexures.
   • Weeping, oozing or crusted lesions rarely present.
4. **Adult phase** (> 20 years)
   Atopic dermatitis usually resolves in adulthood but the hands, face, neck and rarely diffuse areas of skin with dry lesions may be involved:
   • Only 10% of infantile and childhood cases persist into adulthood.

• Atopic dermatitis cannot be cured but various measures can control it:
  - Avoid provoking factors.
  - Reduce dryness and pruritus by using emollients on wet skin.
  - For acutely inflamed and weeping skin use open wet compresses.
  - For sub-acute or chronic lesions→ topical corticosteroids are the mainstay.
  - For resistant or widespread plaques → topical corticosteroids under occlusion.
  - Tar preparations → vaso constrictive, astringent, disinfectant and antipruritus.

  Antibiotic therapy for secondary infections.

Treatment

General Therapeutic Guidelines

The most important aeroallergens in atopy are:

• House dust.
• House dust mite.
• Pollen (tree/grass/weed).
• Animal dander (cat/dog).
• Moulds.

It is generally believed that they should be avoided. In fact for house dust mite allergens, elimination has indeed been proved to have a beneficial effect on the course of atopic dermatitis. Contact with these allergens is prevented by use of dust mite proof (Goretex) covers for mattresses and pillows, wet-mopping floors and avoiding drugs (especially in bedrooms).

Several investigators emphasize the aetiological role of food allergens in atopic dermatitis and note improvement after an elimination diet. Common food allergens implicated in atopic dermatitis are:

• Milk.
• Egg whites.
• Peanuts.
• Soyabeans.
• Tree nuts.

- Fish.
- Shellfish.
- Wheat.

It is accepted that with increasing age, the importance of food allergens rapidly decreases. The frequency of positive reactions to aero-allergens increases with age whereas the frequency of positive reactions to food allergens decreases with age.

Three components of treatment:

- **Steroids.**
- **Emollient.**
- **Anti-Pruritic Agents.**

Others:

- Tacrolimus.
- UVB therapy.
- EFA.
- Cyclosporine.

Algorithm for treatment of atopic dermatitis

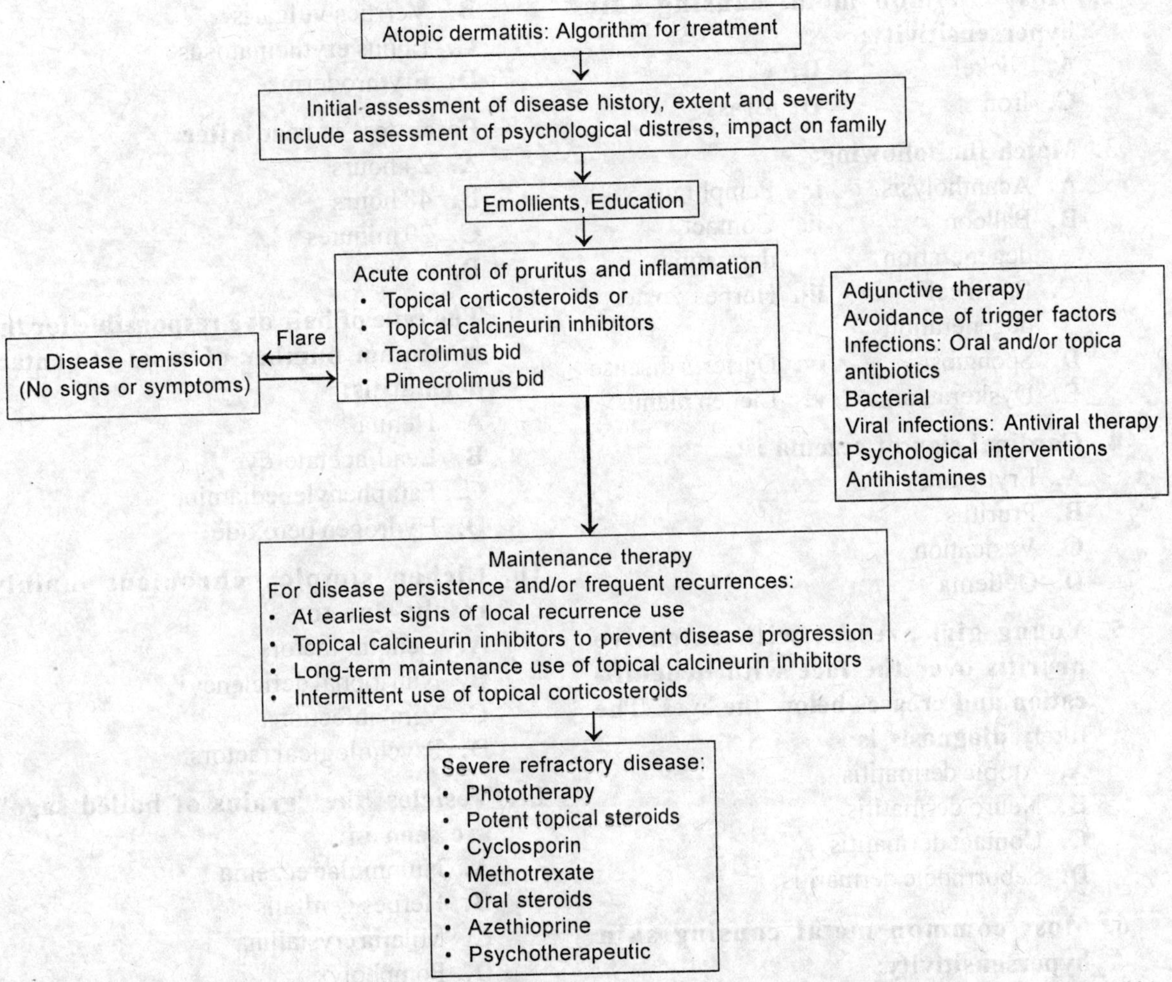

The evidence of the safety and efficacy of pimecrolimus and derived from studies primarily in patients with mild-to-moderate atopic dermatitis, tacrolimus data was derived from moderate-to-severe patients

MULTIPLE CHOICE QUESTIONS

1. A common plant in India which causes contact dermatitis is:
A. Parthenium
B. Asparagus
C. Claviceps purpura
D. Aspergillus

2. Most common metal causing skin hypersensitivity:
A. Nickel B. Cu
C. Iron D. Brass

3. Match the following:

A.	Acantholysis	i.	Pemphigus
B.	Balloon degeneration	ii.	Contact dermatitis
C.	Basal cell degeneration	iii.	Herpes zoster
D.	Spongiosis	iv.	Darier's disease
E.	Dyskeratosis	v.	Lichen planus

4. Cardinal sign of eczema is:
A. Erythema
B. Pruritus
C. Vesication
D. Oedema

5. Young girl present with extensive pruritis over the face with lichenification and creases below the eyes. The likely diagnosis is:
A. Atopic dermatitis
B. Neuro dermatitis
C. Contact dermatitis
D. Seborrhoeic dermatitis

6. Most common metal causing skin hypersensitivity:
A. Nickel
B. Cu
C. Iron
D. Brass

7. Deck chair sign is positive in:
A. Lichen planus
B. Verruca vulgaris
C. Lupus erythematosus
D. Erythroderma

8. Patch test is read after:
A. 24 hours
B. 48 hours
C. 20 minutes
D. 1 week

9. The type of hair dye responsible for the maximum number of cases of contact dermatitis:
A. Henna
B. Lead acetate dye
C. Paraphenylenediamine
D. Hydrogen peroxide

10. Lichen simplex chronicus mainly results due to:
A. Genetic factors
B. Nutritional deficiency
C. Viral infections
D. Psychological factors

11. Vesicles like "grains of boiled sago" are seen in:
A. Nummular eczema
B. Herpes genitalis
C. Milaria crystallina
D. Pompholyx

1 A 2 A 3 A(i),B(iii), C(v),D(ii), E(iv) 4 C 5 A 6 A 7 D 8 B 9 C
10 D 11 D

12. Sailor's skin result from:
- **A.** Chronic solar dermatitis
- **B.** Ichthyosis vulgaris
- **C.** Atopic dermatitis
- **D.** Seborrhoeic dermatitis

13. All true of berloque dermatitis *except*:
- **A.** Caused by beugamot oil contained in perfumes
- **B.** Wave lengths between 290-320 nn are involved
- **C.** Deep brown pigmentation along the trickling of perfume
- **D.** The pigmentation fades after weeks or months
- **E.** Disorders of keratinization

14. Following are common sites for Lichen simplex chronicus *except*:
- **A.** Dorsum of foot
- **B.** Nape of neck
- **C.** Front of legs
- **D.** The scalp

15. Which of the following condition is an absolute indication for the use of corticosteroids?
- **A.** Exfoliative dermatitis
- **B.** Irritant dermatitis
- **C.** Sub acute dermatitis
- **D.** Light dermatitis

16. Out of following sites, Lichen simplex chronicus most often affects:
- **A.** Chest
- **B.** Back
- **C.** Scrotum
- **D.** Face

17. Cheiropompholyx is most common:
- **A.** Palms
- **B.** Nape of neck
- **C.** Soles
- **D.** Abdomen

12 A 13 B 14 D 15 A 16 C 17 A

Chapter 10

Atopic Dermatitis

It is an eczema characterised by intense itching and relapsing course in infants and children with a personal and family history of atopy. It is a common skin disorder.

- 10% of infants are affected.
- 80% have associated asthma and rhinitis.
- 70% have family history of atopy.

AD has three phases:

Infantile Phase

Upto 2 years—Characterised clinically by:

- Intense itching.
- Dry skin.
- Ill defined erythematous patches on the cheeks.
- Dry scaly erythematous plaques on the extensor aspect of limbs along with papulovesicles with oozing and crusting.

Childhood Phase

Between 3 and 11 years—Phase of flexural involvement characterised by involvement of cubital and popliteal fossa. Lesions tend to be more dry.

Adolescent/Adult Phase

Between 12 and 23 years—Involvement of face, neck, flexures and upper trunk is characteristic. Excoriations and lichenification due to scratching are present.

Course of atopic dermatitis is marked by exacerbations and remissions. Provocative factors include—aeroallergens, food, microbial organisms, sweating, climate and physicic stress.

Treatment includes—avoidance of provocative factors, avoidance of high protein diet, regular use if emolients, topical steroids and antihistaminics.

MULTIPLE CHOICE QUESTIONS

1. A 25-year-old man presents with recurrent episodes of flexural eczema, contact urticaria recurrent skin infections and severe abdominal cramps and diarrhoea upon taking sea foods. He is suffering from:

A. Seborrheic dermatitis
B. Atopic dermatitis
C. Airborne contact dermatitis
D. Nummular dermatitis

2. The metabolic explanation to atopic dermatitis is:

A. Hyperuricemia
B. Deranged fatty acid metabolism
C. Vitamin D deficiency
D. Reduced cholesterol synthesis

3. "White dermographism" is a characteristic feature of:

A. Atopic dermatitis
B. Contact dermatitis
C. Seborrheic dermatitis
D. Lichen planus

1 B 2 B 3 A

Chapter 11

Sexually Transmitted Diseases

CLASSIFICATION OF COMMON SEXUALLY TRANSMITTED DISEASES AGENTS

1. Bacteria:
   - Neisseria gonorrhea.
   - Chlamydia trachomatis.
   - Treponema pallidum.
   - Haemophilus ducreyi.
   - Calymmatobacterium granulomatosis.
   - Ureaplasma urealyticum.
   - Gardnerella vaginalis.
   - Shigella spp.
   - Campylobacter spp.
   - Group B streptococcus.
2. Viruses:
   - Herpes simplex virus.
   - Human papillomavirus.
   - Poxvirus.
   - Hepatitis B virus.
   - Human immunodeficiency virus.
3. Protozoa:
   - Trichomonas vaginalis.
   - Griardia lamblia.
   - Entamoeba histolytica.
4. Fungi:
   - Candida albicans.
5. Ectoparasites:
   - Phthirus pubis.
   - Sarcoptes scabiei.

SYPHILIS

Causative organism is Treponema pallidum - incubation period of 3 weeks, with a range from 9 to 90 days, risk of transmission ranges - one third of sexual partners with a single exposure to early syphilis become infected. Late disease is generally associated with minimal risk of transmission.

The primary lesion is a painless chancre at the site of inoculation. Five percent of these chancres are extragenital, lesion begins as an erythematous macule that ulcerates within days. This ulcer is normally solitary and indurated with a nonpurulent, clean base and yellow-gray exudates. Several days later, a painless, bilateral, regional lymphadenopathy often results. **The majority of primary chancres heal within 6 weeks of presentation**. 50% of untreated syphilis infections progress to the second stage, whereas the other 50% enter latency.

The secondary stage of syphilis typically begins 6 to 8 weeks after the onset of the primary lesion. Although the primary lesion is localized to the site of inoculation, secondary syphilis results from hematogenous dissemination and thus presents with widespread manifestations. **Constitutional symptoms, such as fever, malaise, or generalized lymphadenopathy, are common.** The skin is most frequently

STD	Syphilis	Chancroid	LGV	GI	Herpes Genital	Genital Warts	Gonorrhea
Organism	Treponema pallidum	Haemophilus ducreyi	Chlamydia trachomatis (L_1, L_2, L_3)	Calymmatobact granulomatis	Herpes simplex virus 1 + 2	Human papiloma virus (6,11,16,18, 30-32,42,43, 51-55 etc.)	Neisseria gonorrhoea
Clinical Feature	IP→ 9–90 days	2-7 days	3-30 days	8-80 days	3-12 days	Few weeks→ months	2-10 days
Morphology	Single non-tender necrotic, indurated, clean ulcer, oozes serum	Multiple, necrotic, small, non-tender, indurated ulcers with undermined edges, red halo	Transient, herpetiform, spontaneously healing vesicular	Single, beefy, non-indurated, non-tender, granutomatous bleeds on touch	Multiple, grouped, superficial vesicles, erosions with serpiginous margins (poly cyclic)	Usually multiple vegetative, verrueous, dry, grayish white or pinkish soft papillomatous projections	Urethritis + copious, thick yellow, purulent discharge per urethra
Inguinal LAPathy	Rubbery, discrete, mobile, non-tender	Inguinal bubo, unilateral uniocular, tender	Inguinal bubo, unilateral in 2/3 multilocular, tender	—	Tender LAP	—	—
Constitutional symptoms	Generally absent	—	Marked	—	±	—	Fever malaise headache
Lab. Dx	Dark ground microscopy Serology– VORL, TPI, FTA-abs, TPHA, etc.	Scrape smear (Gram stain) → School of fish (gram –ve) —	— Hyperglobulinemia Micro immunofluorescence	Donovan bodies in mononuclear cells on Giemsa stained tissue	Tzanch smear → multinuclear Giant cells Viral culture DIF, E/M	Clinical, H/path, typing, PCR, Nucleic acid hybridization	Gram stained smear → Gram (–) diplococci + Culture for confirmation
Treatment of choice	Inj. Benzathine Penicillin 2.4 mega units AST I/M	Erythromycin P/O 500 mg QID × 7 d	Tetracycline 500 mg QID × 2-3 wks	Streptomycin I/M 2 g in 2 div. doses × 10-20 d or tetracycline	Tab Acyclovir 200 mg × 5 times a day × 5 days + Symptomatic treatment	25% Podophyllin local application (PODOWART)	Inj. Procaine Penicillin 4.8 mega units I/M AST + Ig Probenoid
Other drugs used	Doxycycline PO Tetracycline Erythromycin (pregnant females)	Ceftriaxone I/M Tremitho/sulphamethox Amox + clavalanic acid	Doxycycline Erythromycin Sulphamethoxazole	Co-trimoxazole	—	Podophylotoxin (0.5% –self application Cauterization LASER etc.)	Ceftriaxone IM, Sprotinomycin IM, Ciprofloxacin PO

affected, 80% of patients demonstrating **cutaneous** involvement. The second stage is the most contagious period of syphilis. A generalized macular, maculopapular or papulosquamous rash often appears. Pink macules to (the more common) dusky red, nonpruritic scaling papules present. Lesions have a predilection for palms and soles. Papular involvement of the scalp may lead to patchy syphilitic alopecia.

Condyloma latum often occurs when the papular eruption is located in moist intertriginous areas, such as the buttocks, groin, labia or inner thighs. Opposition of the moist surfaces causes maceration of the papule, forming broad flat-topped lesions. These lesions are the most infectious variety of secondary syphilis.

Thirty percent to 50% of all patients with secondary syphilis also develop mucous membrane involvement. The most common manifestation is the syphilitic sore throat, and the second most common is the mucous patch.

Without treatment, secondary syphilis spontaneously resolves and enters latency. Latent syphilis may occur between the first and second stages or the second and third stages. This period is characterized by positive serologies without signs or symptoms of disease. Although the causative organism continues to multiply in this stage, patients may remain asymptomatic for life. **Only one third of untreated cases progress to tertiary syphilis. The latent stage is divided into early and late periods. Infection of less than 1 year as early latent disease,** which is considered infectious. Meanwhile, that which is greater than 1 year is described as late latent disease, which is considered noninfectious. The World Health Organization has established a dividing line of 2 years between these stages.

Tertiary syphilis may present many years after inoculation and most commonly affects the cutaneous, neural, and cardiovascular systems. Two different types of **cutaneous** lesions may arise:

1. **Nodular or noduloulcerative lesions** are small, firm, nonpruritic and painless and predominantly affect the back, face and arms. These lesions have the potential for ulceration with resultant scarring.
2. **Gummas** are painless, deep granulomatous lesions, normally originating from subcutaneous tissue. Predominant locations include the face, scalp, calf, sternum and sternoclavicular area, typically heal with retractile scarring.

The diagnosis of syphilis is usually based on serology. The primary chancre of syphilis, however, may be present for 1 to 3 weeks before serologies become positive. Therefore, it is imperative to perform a dark-field examination or fluorescent microscopy of lesional exudate to visualize the spirochete directly in primary syphilis. screening is first performed with the nontreponemal tests, Venereal Disease Research Laboratory (VDRL) and rapid plasma reagin (RPR).

With late syphilis, the non-treponemal antibody titers do not always decrease as expected. False-positive results may occur for multiple reasons, including collagen vascular disease, advancing age, chronic liver disease, narcotic drug use, various acute infections such as herpes, and numerous chronic infections such as tuberculosis or HIV. Because of **the lower specificity of these tests, positive results should be confirmed with the more precise treponemal tests, fluorescent treponemal antibody absorption test (FTA-ABS) and microhemagglutination assay** for T. pallidum (MTA-TP). Treponemal tests do not correspond to disease activity, and they normally remain reactive indefinitely despite effective treatment.

The treatment for primary, secondary, and early latent syphilis is a single intramuscular dose of benzathine penicillin G 2.4 million

units. A four-fold decrease in antibody titers should be evident at 3 months to ensure successful therapy. There is a risk of treatment failure in 5% to 10% and retreatment for patients without neurosyphilis is recommended as three weekly injections of benzathine penicillin G. Late latent and tertiary syphilis are both treated with three intramuscular injections of benzathine penicillin G 2.4 million units given at weekly intervals.

Patients who are allergic to penicillin may be given alternative treatments, such as doxycycline, tetracycline, or erythromycin, or they may undergo desensitization to penicillin. patients may experience an acute febrile reaction within 24 hours, called the Jarisch-Herxheimer reaction. This complication includes headache and myalgia, among other symptoms, and is more prevalent among patients with primary syphilis.

Interactions between syphilis and HIV - Syphilis and other ulcerative STDs are implicated as facilitators of both HIV transmission and acquisition because they may provide a favorable portal of entry for the virus. HIV may cause false-positive nontreponemal serologies in the absence of syphilis. Therefore dark-field examination or biopsy may be necessary in equivocal cases. extended follow-up is necessary to ensure complete resolution.

CHANCROID

Chancroid caused by the organism Haemophilus ducreyi. Incubation period—3 to 7 days. The characteristic ulcer is friable, soft, and nonindurated, with ragged undermined margins and surrounding erythema. The lesion is often covered with a gray or yellow necrotic exudates. **After 1 week 50% of patients develop inguinal lymphadenopathy, which is typically painful and unilateral.** A suppurative bubo occurs in 25% of all patients, which may spontaneously rupture and discharge thick pus. This results in a large, deep inguinal ulceration. autoinoculation may result in the classic kissing lesions.

Chancroid may have a variety of presentations:

1. The **classic form** consists of ulcers ranging in diameter from 3 to 20 mm with multiple lesions caused by autoinoculation.
2. **Dwarf chancroid** presents as single or multiple herpetiform ulcerations with or without inguinal lymphadenopathy.
3. **Transient chancroid** has an ulcer that rapidly resolves in 4 to 6 days and is followed by suppurative inguinal lymphadenopathy in 10 to 20 days.
4. The **follicular form** consists of ulcerations in the pilar apparatus in hair-bearing areas.
5. **Giant chancroid** presents as multiple small ulcerations that rapidly expand and coalesce to form a single, large destructive lesion. This form is often associated with inguinal bubo formation.
6. **Phagedenic chancroid** results in widespread necrosis and extensive soft tissue destruction of the genitalia. Finally, pseudogranuloma inguinale a form of chancroid that closely resembles granuloma inguinale.

The **diagnosis of chancroid is based on clinical presentation,** which may be accurate in only 33% to 53% of cases. Defmitive diagnosis is made with culture of the causative organism. Even under optimal conditions, culture has an accuracy of less than 80% and is not sensitive enough to detect all cases.

A painful ulceration with tender inguinal lymphadenopathy is suggestive of chancroid, whereas an association with suppurative adenopathy is almost pathognomonic. If diagnosis must rely on clinical morphology, it is important to perform serologic and dark-field examinations for syphilis and culture for herpes, to rule out common causes of genital ulceration.

Treatment for chancroid consists of a single 1-g dose of oral azithromycin, one 250 mg intramuscular injection of ceftriaxone,

or 500 mg oral erythromycin base four times per day for 7 days. Alternative regimens include oral amoxicillin-clavulanic acid 500/125 mg three times per day for 7 days or oral ciprofloxacin 500 mg twice a day for 3 days.

Ciprofloxacin is contraindicated in children less than 17 years old and pregnant or lactating women. With treatment, ulcerations should resolve within 1 to 2 weeks. Larger fluctuant nodes heal rather slowly and have a risk of spontaneous rupture, resulting in chronic ulcers and tissue loss. For this reason, prophylactic aspiration or incision and drainage is advised.

Coinfection with HIV and chancroid may result in significantly altered clinical features. These include large ulcerations, extragenital lesions, less prominent regional adenopathy, and delayed healing with standard therapy.

LYMPHOGRANULOMA VENEREUM

The responsible organism for lymphogranuloma venereum (LGV) is Chlamydia trachomatis, immunotypes L_1, L_2, and L_3. The incubation period for this organism is normally 10 to 14 days with a range of 3 days to 6 weeks. Immediately thereafter, the **primary** lesion develops as a small painless papule, which erodes to form a shallow ulceration. This transient lesion heals within a few days and is appreciated only in a minority of patients.

Within 2 to 6 weeks after the primary lesion, the second stage develops. This period is known as the inguinal stage because it produces inflammation of the inguinal or femoral lymph nodes. These nodes are painful, swollen and most commonly unilateral. They may develop into suppurative buboes with spontaneous rupture in one third of the cases. 20% of patients have enlargement of both inguinal and femoral nodes, which results in an indentation or groove at the inguinal ligament. This groove sign is pathognomonic for LGV. Constitutional symptoms are rather common in the second stage and may include fever, malaise, arthralgia, myalgia and anorexia.

Without treatment, the chronic lymphangitis of LGV may result in fistulas, sinus tracts, and ulcerations, which lead to extensive scarring, strictures, ischemia, and tissue necrosis. Chronic lymphedema and lymphatic obstruction may occasionally result in elephantiasis years later. Elephantiasis of the female genitalia is called esthiomene and leads to fibrotic labial thickening.

The third stage of LGV is described as the genitoanorectal stage. Although the second stage is more common in men, the third stage more frequently affects homosexuals and women who engage in receptive anal intercourse. Proctocolitis first begins, with symptoms of fever, tenesmus, rectal pain, and pruritus. **Hyperplasia of perirectal lymphatic tissue results in lymphorrhoids, which are similar to hemorrhoids.** This stage is also associated with rectal strictures, perirectal abscesses and fistulas.

Definitive diagnosis of LGV is made with cultural isolation of the organism. This method, however, has a recovery rate of less than 30%. Therefore, diagnosis is based on serology associated with appropriate clinical findings. A complement fixation titer (LGV-CF) of greater than 1:16 is strongly suggestive of this diagnosis. Serology is normally positive within 2 weeks of onset. **Antibody titers do not necessarily correspond with disease activity and may not decline after treatment, as in syphilis.**

The preferred treatment for LGV is oral doxycycline 100 mg twice daily for 21 days. Alternative treatments are oral sulfisoxazole or erythromycin, with erythromycin as the drug of choice for pregnant women. The dosage for either drug is 500 mg four times per day for 21 days. Prophylactic aspiration or incision and drainage of fluctuant lymph nodes may also be necessary.

GRANULOMA INGUINALE

Granuloma inguinale, or donovanosis, is a result of **infection with Calymmatobacterium granulomatis**. After an incubation period of 8 days to 12 weeks, single or multiple subcutaneous nodules develop at the site of inoculation.

These lesions erode to form painless ulcerations that have clean, friable bases and distinct rolled margins. **True inguinal lymphadenopathy does not occur,** although a few patients have associated swelling and ulceration in the inguinal area because of infection around the lymph node. This entity is described as a **pseudobubo.** Without treatment, granuloma inguinale does not tend to heal spontaneously but leads to progressive destruction of the genitalia, with extensive scarring and fibrosis.

Multiple variants of granuloma inguinale exist:

1. **The ulcerovegetative or ulcerogranulomatous form is the most common variant,** producing large, extensive ulcerations.
2. **Nodular granuloma** inguinale consists of soft, red nodules, which then erode to form ulcers.
3. The **hypertrophic form** produces large vegetating masses that may resemble condylomata acuminata.
4. Lastly, **cicatricial** granuloma inguinale is a rare form associated with expanding scar tissue formation.

Isolation of C granulomatis is difficult and impractical. Hence diagnosis is based on direct visualization of the intracytoplasmic Donovan bodies (safety pin-shaped organisms). This is achieved with Giemsa or Wright staining of tissue smears or skin biopsy specimens.

The standard treatment for granuloma inguinale is either oral tetracycline 500 mg four times per day for 2 to 3 weeks or oral doxycycline 100 mg twice a day for 2 to 3 weeks. Many strains of granuloma inguinale worldwide are now resistant to tetracycline and its derivatives. Alternative therapy includes oral trimethoprim-sulfamethoxazole 160/800 mg twice a day for 2 to 3 weeks or oral erythromycin 500 mg four times per day for 2 to 3 weeks.

GENITAL HERPES

Genital herpes has traditionally been **associated with herpes simplex virus type 2 (HSV-2).** 30% of these infections are due to HSV-1 as a result of orogenital sex.

The average incubation period for HSV is 7 to 10 days, with a range of 2 to 21 days. After incubation, the primary lesion arises, comprised multiple, small, grouped vesicles on an erythematous base.

After several days, these vesicles erode to form **painful shallow ulcers with eventual crusting.** Constitutional symptoms and inguinal lymphadenopathy may also accompany the primary lesion. **The adenopathy may be tender, yet is not fluctuant**. Untreated the lesion persists for an average of 3 weeks, with a peak in the severity of symptoms at 1.5 weeks. Thirty percent of patients with genital herpes have lesions in nongenital locations, such as the thighs or buttocks.

Recurrent lesions are less severe and have a shorter course of 7 to 10 days. often preceded by a pruritic prodromal period of 1 to 4 days. **Genital HSV-2 infections typically recur earlier and more frequently than those of HSV-1.** Most patients with HSV-2 are likely to experience recurrent disease. Men have a 20% greater frequency of recurrences than women. Triggers are implicated in reactivation, including local trauma from intercourse or masturbation, menstruation, and psychological factors such as stress.

Asymptomatic shedding is an important factor for the transmission of herpes and is responsible for 70% to 80% of new cases. Women have a significantly higher risk of acquiring herpes than men.

Diagnosis of genital herpes is often based on clinical presentation but should be confirmed by viral culture, if possible. Other means of diagnosis are visualization of multinucleated giant cells on Tzanck or Papanicolaou smears, viral antigen and DNA detection tests, and electron microscopy. Serologic assays are significantly less sensitive and less specific than viral isolation and are not useful for the diagnosis of genital herpes.

The **treatment** for primary episodes of herpes is oral acyclovir 200 mg five times per day for 7 to 10 days. Recurrences may be addressed by long term suppressive therapy viz. 400 mg TDS for 6 months to 1 year.

Episodic patient-initiated therapy is effective if taken during the prodromal period or within 2 days of lesion formation. Acyclovir 200 mg five times per day, 400 mg three times per day, or 800 mg twice a day is given for 5 days. Side effects of continuous acyclovir treatment include nausea, diarrhea, headache and a rash. Adverse effects are usually of minimal severity and decrease with time.

Valacyclovir is a dependable alternative to acyclovir. Valacyclovir is a prodrug, which is almost completely converted to acyclovir after absorption from the intestine. Thus, it carries the same safety record and efficacy, while providing improved absorption and less frequent dosing. The treatment regimen includes 500 mg twice a day for 5 days for episodic therapy and 500 mg once to twice a day for suppressive therapy. Famciclovir is another treatment alternative for herpes.

The **interactions between herpes and HIV** are well documented. Immunosuppression from HIV infection may promote severe, chronic, and highly infectious ulcerations with herpes. Although ulcers in healthy individuals resolve within a few weeks, they may persist for several months in patients with HIV.

The treatment of herpes in HIV-positive patients remains the same as for HIV-negative individuals. Acyclovir resistance has been reported to occur in 2.9% of immunocompromised patients on suppressive therapy. In these cases, foscarnet has often been effective, yet it is associated with nephrotoxicity and frequent relapses after discontinuation of treatment.

GENITAL WARTS

As in herpes, only a **minority of human papillomavirus (HPV) infections appear to result in noticeable lesions.** Anogenital warts, also known as **condylomata acuminata**, are benign growths that are most commonly associated with HPV types 6 or 11. These warts typically present as soft, flesh-colored papules that may progress to a cauliflower-like mass. Multiple clustered lesions are typically present, yet a solitary wart may occasionally occur. **The most common locations in men are the glans, edge of the corona, prepuce, shaft, frenulum, and scrotum. Sites of predilection in women include the labia, perineum, clitoris, and fourchette.** The majority of patients who present with genital warts also have subclinical HPV infection, often including many other HPV types. Therefore **all affected women should be screened for cervical intraepithelial neoplasia.** Untreated, condylomata acuminata may spontaneously regress, enlarge, or remain unchanged. Rarely the warts themselves may undergo malignant transformation with time.

The **treatment for genital warts**—Removal of the warts does not eradicate the virus because the surrounding areas are usually subclinically infected.

Podophyllotoxin 0.5% solution or gel is a method of home treatment that is a useful first-line therapy for responsible patients. Podophyllin 10% to 25% in tincture of benzoin is a useful first-line office treatment. If the warts persist after six tries, another method should be considered, such as cryotherapy or electrocautery.

Trichloroacetic acid 80-90% may be applied once weekly. If lesions persist after six applications, another therapy should be considered. This therapy may be applied during pregnancy when podophyllin is contraindicated.

Electrocautery and electrodesiccation are used for recalcitrant warts and typically require one to two treatments. HPV DNA can be inhaled.

Vaginal warts should be treated with cryotherapy or trichloroacetic acid, whereas warts of the urethral meatus should be treated with cryotherapy or podophyllin.

GENITAL SCABIES

Although scabies can be transmitted nonsexually, particularly in children, it is commonly **sexually** acquired in adults. The **causal ectoparasite is Sarcoptes scabiei** or the itch mite. Prolonged skin contact between individuals is a common mode of transmission. The female mite burrows into the skin to feed and lay her **eggs, which hatch in 3 to 4 days and evolve into adult mites in 14 to 17 days.** The clinical symptoms are a result of a hypersensitivity reaction to the mite antigens. In a patient without previous exposure it may take 4 to 8 weeks to begin. In a previously exposed person, symptoms normally develop within a few days.

Clinical manifestations begin with a small burrow, which appears as an elongated papule. The mite may sometimes be visualized in early disease as a tiny dot at the end of the burrow. Burrows are found on interdigital webs of the hands and on the glans penis. All lesions are associated with intense pruritus, which is characteristically worse at night.

Diagnosis is often clinical, followed by empiric treatment. Different medications are currently recommended.

1. **Permethrin 5% cream** is applied to the entire body from the neck down. It should be washed off 8 to 14 hours after application. This therapy can be used in young children and pregnant women.
2. **Lindane 1% lotion** (1-oz dose) or cream (30-g dose) should be thinly applied to the entire body from the neck down and washed off after 8 hours. Central nervous system toxicity has been reported from overuse cannot be used in children less than 2 years old or pregnant or lactating women.
3. **Crotomiton 10%** is considered an alternative treatment. It does not appear equally effective. It should be applied from the neck down on 2 consecutive nights. Twenty-four hours after the second application, the body is then washed.

Pruritus may continue for several weeks after treatment.

To prevent reinfestation, all close contacts of the patient, particularly sexual and bed partners, should be simultaneously treated.

HIV-infected individuals with immunocompromise have an increased risk for **Norwegian (crusted) scabies. Crusted scabies carries a significant risk of secondary bacterial infection** and bacterial septicemia. This form of scabies responds more slowly to conventional therapy and often requires multiple applications. Oral administration of the antiparasitic drug **ivermectin is currently under investigation** for scabies therapy in both normal and immunocompromised hosts.

Pelvic Inflammatory Disease (PID)

PID comprises a spectrum of inflammatory disorders of the female upper genital tract, including any combination of endometritis, salpingitis, tubo-ovarian abscess and pelvic peritonitis. It may be of the chronic (caused by M. tuberculosis) or acute PID (caused by sexual pathogens). This section will be dealing with acute PID

- **Cervical pathogens:** N. gonorrhea, Chlamydia trachomatis.
- **Vaginal microorganisms:** Anaerobic bacteria (e.g. Prevotella, Peptostreptococcus), H

influenzae, Gardnerella vaginalis, Mycoplasma hominis and Ureaplasma urealyticum

Symptoms and Signs

Wide variations is symptoms in women depending on the pathogen and the site of pathology:

- Malodorous, yellowish vaginal discharge.
- Midline abdominal pain, abnormal vaginal bleeding (due to endometritis).
- Dyspareunia.
- Lower abdominal and pelvic pain (salpingitis).
- Fever, nausea vomiting, abdominal tenderness and rigidity (due to peritonitis).

(*Fitz-Hugh-Curtis* syndrome refers to perihepatitis with acute PID caused by gonococcus or chlamydia. Patient presents with pleuritic upper abdominal pain and violin-string adhesions over the liver seen on laparoscopy).

Diagnostic Criteria

Minimum criteria:

- Uterine/adnexal tenderness
- Cervical motion tenderness.

Additional criteria:

- Oral temperature > 101°F.
- Abnormal cervical or vaginal discharge.
- WBC's on saline mount of vaginal discharge.
- Elevated ESR and C-reactive protein.
- Laboratory documentation of cervical infection with *N. gonorrhea or C trachomatis.*

Specific criteria (required only in certain cases):

- Endometrial biopsy showing in certain cases.
- Transvaginal sonography or MRI scan showing tubal abnormalities or tubovarial abscess.
- Laparoscopic findings of PID.

Treatment

- Treatment should be initiated with minimal criteria and needs to cover all the etiological pathogens. Early treatment prevents sequelae.
- Parenteral therapy is given for the initial 24-48 hours and thereafter oral therapy is continued.

Regimens include: IV Cefoxitin plus oral doxycycline (after 24 hours IV drugs stopped and oral doxycycline continued) or IV clindamycin and gentamicin (24 hours) followed by oral doxycycline or IV of loxacin with metronidazole or IV ampicillin plus doxycycline:

- Many sexual contacts (in the preceding 60 days) should be treated.

Bacterial Vaginosis

- Bacterial vaginosis (BV) is a common cause of abnormal vaginal discharge in women of reproductive age.
- It represents a complex change in vaginal flora characterized by a reduction in the prevalence and concentration of hydrogen peroxide producing lactobacilli and increase in the prevalence and concentration of Gardnerella vaginalis; Mobiluncus species; Mycoplasma hominis; anaerobic gram-negative rods belonging to the general Prevotella, Porphyromonas, and bacteriodes; and Peptostreptococcus species.
- **Amsel et al.** Diagnosis requires three or more of the following clinical/diagnostic features:
  - **The presence of (excessive) homogeneous vaginal discharge.**
  - **Elevated vaginal pH > 4.5.**
  - **Positive amine test (Whiff test).**
  - **20% "clue cells" (vaginal epithelial cells adhered to by infective microbes) and typical Gram stain appearance upon microscopy of vaginal secretions including absence of lactobacilli.**

Treatment

- All women who have symptomatic BV disease require treatment.
- Metronidazole 500 mg orally twice a day for 7 days, or Metronidazole gel 0.75% one full applicator (5 g) intravaginally, once a day for 5 days, or Clindamycin cream 2%, one

Table 11.1: Differential diagnoses of vaginal discharge

Profile	*Normal vaginal discharge*	*Candidal vulvovaginitis*	*Trichomonal vaginitis*	*Bacterial vaginosis*
Etiology	Lactobacillus	Candida spp. and other yeasts	Trichomonas vaginitis	Associated with G. vaginalis; anaerobic bacteria, and Mycoplasma hominis
Symptoms	None	Vulvar Pruritus and/or irritation; external Dysuria, increased	Profuse discharge, often malodorous; external Dysuria and genital irritation often present	Malodorous, increased discharge (commonly present at the introitus)
Discharge amount	Variable; usually scant	Scant to moderate white	Profuse	Moderate to profuse
Color	Clear or white	White	White, yellow or green	White or gray
Consistency	Nonhomogenous, focculant	Clumped, "Cheesy" adherent exudative plaques < 4.5	Homogeneous, watery, often frothy	Homogeneous, uniformly coating vaginal walls
pH	Usually < 4.5	<4.5	Usually > 5.0	Usually > 4.5
Amine odor with 10% KOH	None	None	Usually present	Present
Associated inflammatory signs	None	Erythema, edema and/or erosions of vagina or external genitalia, vulvar dermatitis common	Erythema of vaginal mucosa, introitus; occasional cervical petechiae; vulvar dermatitis	None
Microscopy of discharge	Normal epithelial cells; lactobacilli predominate	Leukocytes, epithelial cells, yeast, mycelia, pseudomycelia seen	Leukocytes, motile trichomonads seen	Clue cells; rare leukocytes; lactobacilli outnumbered by mixed flora

applicator intravaginally 4 days are recommended treatments.

- Alternatively, patient may be treated with Metronidazole 2 g orally in a single dose, Clindamycin 300 mg orally twice a day for 7 days, or Clindamycin ovules 100 g intravaginally once at bed time for 3 days (Table 11.1).

PEDICULOSIS PUBIS

Pediculosis pubis is predominantly a **sexually** transmitted infestation, particularly in the young, single, **sexually** active population. The **causative ectoparasite is Phthirus pubis, or the crab louse,** which inhabits only humans. These lice can survive off their host for upto 24 hours. direct transmission through skin contact is the primary method for infestation. After an incubation period of 1 week, the eggs hatch, with maturation of the lice over the following 2 weeks. **Cutaneous** manifestations may not be evident but include inflammatory papules, wheals, or blue spots located at feeding sites.

Lindane 1% shampoo can be applied to affected areas only and washed off after 4 minutes. This treatment is contraindicated in children less than 2 years old and in pregnant or lactating women. Alternatively, either permethrin 1% cream or pyrethrins 0.3% with piperonyl butoxide 3% may be applied to affected areas and washed off after 10 minutes. None of these treatments should be applied to the eyes.

MULTIPLE CHOICE QUESTIONS

1. All of the following strategies are effective in preventing mother to child transmission of HIV, *except*:
A. Zidovudine to mother and baby
B. Vaginal cleansing before delivery
C. Stopping breastfeeding
D. Elective caesarean section

2. A 30-year-old male patient has a large, spreading and exuberant ulcer with bright red granulation tissue over the glans penis. There was no lymph-adenopathy. The most likely causative organism is:
A. Treponema pallidum
B. Herpes simplex virus type 1
C. Herpes simplex virus type 2
D. Calymmatobacterium granulomatis

3. Which of the following is the drug of first choice for non-gonococcal urethritis?
A. Ceftriaxone
B. Ciprofloxacin
C. Doxycycline
D. Minocycline

4. Treatment of early latent syphillis is:
A. Benzathine penicillin 2.4 MU stat
B. Cotrimoxazole for 1 month
C. Doxycycline for 1 week
D. Crystallin penicillin for 2 weeks

5. Bullous and vesicular lesions in syphilis are seen in:
A. Primary stage
B. Secondary
C. Tertiary
D. Congenital syphilis

6. Earliest skin lesion in congenital syphilis is:
A. Rhagades
B. Syphilitic pemphigus
C. Papules
D. Roseolar rash

7. Pseudo-bubo is seen in:
A. Chancriod
B. Secondary syphilis
C. Donavanosis
D. Gonorrhoea

8. The test to become positive first in syphilis is:
A. VDRL
B. FTAABS
C. TPHA
D. TPI

9. Cutaneous lesions secondary to gonococcal bacteraemia are typically:
A. Haemorrhagic vesiculopustular
B. Purpura
C. Punched out ulcers
D. Tender nodules

10. All of the following are true regarding Jarisch-Herxheimer reaction *except*:
A. It is due to sudden massive destruction of spirochaetes by drugs
B. Most likely to occur in early syphilis
C. Usually begins within the first 24 hours of treatment
D. Manifested by vesicular-bullous lesions

1 C 2 D 3 C 4 A 5 D 6 D 7 C 8 B 9 A 10 D

11. A person develops arthritis, conjunctivitis and urethritis 3 weeks after sexual exposure, diagnosis is:
A. Gonococcal infection
B. Reiter's disease
C. LGV
D. Complicated herpes genitalis

12. Chancre-redux is:
A. Recurrence of primary sore at its original site
B. Any lesion at the site of healed primary lesion
C. Primary chancre at extragenital site
D. Another name for soft sore

13. Balanitis is not a feature of:
A. Reiter's disease
B. Balanitis xerotica obliterans
C. Plasma cell Balanitis of zoon
D. Bowen's disease

14. Which of the following conditions is most likely to be associated with a vaginal pH of 4?
A. Atrophic vaginitis
B. Candidal vaginitis
C. Trichomonas vaginitis
D. Gardnerella vaginitis

15. The "sign of groove" is seen in:
A. Syphilis
B. LGV
C. Chancroid
D. Gonorrhoea

16. Hutchinson's triad is seen in:
A. Congenital syphilis
B. Adult syphilis
C. Malignant melanoma
D. Herpes zoster

17. BO sign is positive in:
A. Congenital syphilis
B. Primary syphilis
C. Secondary syphilis
D. Cardiovascular syphilis

18. Treatment of choice for acute gonococcal infection in a male patient is:
A. Inj Ceftriaxone 250 mg IM AST once
B. Inj Ceftriaxone 250 mg IM AST once *and* Cap Doxycyline 100 mg BD × 7 days
C. Tb norfloxacin 400 mg twice daily × 10 days
D. Tb norfloxacin 800 mg once stat

19. School of fish or tram track appearance on Gram stain is characteristic of:
A. Gonococcal infection
B. Haemophilius ducreyi infection
C. Treponema pallidum infection
D. Mycoplasma hominis infection

20. Which of the following STDs is an indication for caesarian section in the mother?
A. Syphilitic chancre
B. Chancroid
C. Genital warts
D. Herpes genitalis

21. Podophyllin application is treatment of choice for:
A. Plantar warts
B. Condyloma lata
C. Condyloma acuminata
D. Plain warts

22. If VDRL is persistently positive, the physician should:
A. Consider latent syphilis if the patient is free of any signs and symptoms
B. Advice 3 injections of benzathine penicillin 2.4 mega units at weekly intervals
C. Order an FTA—Abs test
D. All of the above

11 B 12 A 13 D 14 B 15 B 16 A 17 C 18 B 19 B 20 C 21 C 22 D

23. Apo-eccrine glands are found in:
A. Axilla
B. Peri-umbilical area
C. Perineum
D. Scalp

24. Corneal ulcer in leprosy is most often due to involvements of:
A. Facial nerve
B. Trigeminal nerve
C. Oculocutaneous nerve
D. Optic nerve

25. All true of Neisseria gonorrhea *except*:
A. Some strains produce penicillinase
B. Growson Chacko—Nair medium
C. It can readily infect the pharynx
D. It cannot be cultured from skin lesions

26. Treatment of late latent syphilis is:
A. Single injection of 2.4 units of benzathine penicillin
B. 3 injections of 2.4 mega units of benzathine penicillin on 3 consecutive weeks
C. Single injection of 4.8 mega units of procaine penicillin
D. Resolves on its own, no need for treatment

27. Cutaneous lesions secondary to gonococcal bacteraemia are typically:
A. Haemorrhagic vesiculopustular
B. Purpura
C. Punched out ulcers
D. Tender nodules

28. In syphilis the primary sore or chancre may not develop under following circumstances *except*:
A. Congenital syphilis
B. Infection due to blood transfusion
C. Endemic syphilis
D. Infection due to handling infective materials

29. Syphilis can be transmitted during pregnancy to offspring if mother is having:
A. Primary syphilis
B. Secondary syphilis
C. Early latent syphilis
D. All of the above

30. All of the following are true regarding Jarisch-Herxheimer reaction *except*:
A. It is due to sudden massive destruction of spirochaetes by drugs
B. Most likely to occur in early syphilis
C. Usually begins within the first 24 hours of treatment
D. Manifested by vesicular-bullous lesions

31. If VDRL is persistently positive, the physician should:
A. Consider latent syphilis if the patient is free of any signs and symptoms
B. Advice 3 injections of benzathine penicillin 2.4 mega units at weekly intervals
C. Order an FTA—Abs test
D. All of the above

32. Yaws is caused by:
A. T. caratenum
B. T. pallidum
C. T. pertenue
D. T. canaliculli

33. All are *true* of recurrent herpes genitalis *except*:
A. More than 6 episodes in a year warrants suppressive treatment
B. Even a single recurrence warrants suppressive therapy
C. Causes psychological distress to patient
D. Treatment includes oral acyclovir in suppressive doses for over one year

23 A 24 A 25 D 26 B 27 A 28 D 29 D 30 D 31 C 32 C 33 B

34. **Most reliable test for diagnosing chancroid is:**
A. Clinical features
B. Gram's stained smear
C. ITO test
D. Biopsy

35. **A 20-year-old man developed a small transient genital ulcer 4 weeks after exposure. The regional lymphoid enlarged and become matted together, tender and adherent to the deep tissues. Fever weight loss macular rash and hepato splenomegaly are present. The diagnosis is:**
A. Chancroid
B. LGV
C. Granuloma inguinale
D. Complicated gonorrhea

36. **Incubation period of syphilis is:**
A. 2-3 months
B. 1-3 months
C. 9 days to 3 months
D. 3 weeks to 3 months

37. **The rash of secondary syphilis is usually:**
A. Vesicular
B. Asymptomatic
C. Not seen on palms and soles
D. Not accompanied by lymphadenopathy

38. **Jarisch-Herxheimer reaction is seen most commonly in:**
A. Primary syphilis
B. Secondary syphilis
C. Congenital syphilis
D. Latent syphilis

39. **Treatment of choice for syphilis is:**
A. Tetracycline
B. Erythromycin
C. Short acting penicillin
D. Long acting penicillin

40. **Bullous skin rash is characteristically seen in:**
A. Congenital syphilis
B. Secondary syphilis
C. Primary syphilis
D. Tertiary syphilis

41. **Earliest skin lesions in secondary syphilis is:**
A. Macular/Roseolar
B. Papular
C. Follicular
D. Annular

42. **Earliest skin lesion in congenital syphilis is:**
A. Rhagades
B. Perianal condylomata
C. Bullous rash
D. Papules

43. **Most common site of extragenital chance:**
A. Lip
B. Tongue
C. Tonsil
D. Palate

44. **Most infectious form of syphilis is:**
A. Primary
B. Secondary
C. Tertiary
D. Latent syphilis

45. **Treatment of granuloma inguinale is:**
A. Tetracycline
B. Sulphonamide
C. Streptomycin
D. Penicillin

46. **The venereal disease with the shortest average incubation period is:**
A. Granuloma inguinale
B. Syphilis
C. Chancroid
D. Herpes genitalis

34 B,D 35 B 36 C 37 B 38 B 39 D 40 A 41 A 42 C 43 A 44 B
45 A 46 C

47. **The serological test most suitable for monitoring response to treatment in early syphilis is:**
A. VDRL
B. TPHA
C. FTA-ABS
D. TPI

48. **Multiple painful ulcers without induration are seen in:**
A. Chancroid
B. Granuloma
C. Primary syphilis
D. Lymphogranuloma venerum

49. **A patient with multiple painful necrotic ulcers on glans with tender suppurative unilateral inguinal lymphadenopathy the most likely cause is:**
A. Herpes simplex virus-2
B. Haemophilus ducrei
C. Chlamydia trachomatis
D. Candida albicans

50. **Ito-Reinsterna test is done in:**
A. Leishmaniasis
B. Sarcoidosis
C. LGI
D. Chancroid

51. **The common cause of non-gonococcal urethritis is:**
A. Trichomonas
B. Chlamydiae
C. Mycoplasma
D. Gonococcus

52. **Treatment of non-venereal syphilis is:**
A. Procaine penicillin
B. Benzathine penicillin
C. Tetracycline
D. Sulfonamides

47 A 48 A 49 B 50 D 51 B 52 A

Chapter 12

Cutaneous Vasculitis

Clinical disorder comprising a large spectrum of cutaneous lesions, usually presenting as palpable purpura, characterised by perivascular segmental inflammation, swelling of endothelial cells and fibrinoid necrosis of blood vessel walls.

Incidence—Occurs equally in both sexes and at all ages.

10% cases occur in children.

Etiology includes bacterial infection like β haemolytic streptococci groups A, Mycobacterium leprae, viral infections like hepatitis A,B,C, Herpes simplex, fungal infection like Candida, Protozoal like malaria and helminths schistosomiasis; drugs and chemicals like Insulin, Streptomycin, sulphonamides, thiazides, phenothiazine, oral contraceptive pills, Tamoxifen, Streptokinase insecticides, Petroleum products, Milk protein; Chronic diseases like SLE, Sjögren's, RA, Behcet's, Hypergammaglobulinemia, cryoglobulinemia, Cystic fibrosis, Primary biliary cirrhosis, HIV seropositivity or AIDS; Malignancies like Lymphoproliferative disorders, Hodgkins lymphoma, Mycosis fungoides, Multiple solid tumors of lung, kidney, prostate and breast. Idiopathic causes include Henoch-Schönlein purpura, Urticarial vasculitis , Erythema elevatum diutinum, Nodular vasculitis, Atrophe Blanche, Livedoid vasculitis.

Cutaneous PAN

Clinical Features

1. Palpable purpura.
2. Erythematous macules, papules, blisters, palpable nodules, echymoses, pustules, haemorrhagic vesicles, ulcers, livedo reticularis.
3. Mucous membranes, may have petechial haemorrhages blisters, ulcers.
4. Fever, myalgia, joint pains, headache, malaise
5. Systemic manifestations:
   - **Kidneys**—nephritis with microscopic haematuria and proteinuria, acute and chronic renal failure.
   - **GIT**—pain, nausea, vomiting, diarrhoea, malaena, haematemesis.
   - **Lungs**—asymptomatic, cough and haemoptysis.
   - **Heart**—myocardial angitis, pericarditis.
   - **Nervous system**—headache, diplopia, hypoaesthesia, parasthesia.
   - **Joints**—arthralgia, arthritis.

HENOCH-SCHÖNLEIN PURPURA

Usually occurs in children between 4-8 years of age. Boys are affected more than girls. It often follows streptococcal or respiratory sore throat infection. In 40% cases cutaneous manifestations are preceded by mild fever, headache, joint pains and abdominal pain.

Skin findings include palpable purpura, lesions on lower extremities and buttocks usually sparing the trunks which regress within 10-14 days. Other systemic complaints include GI symptoms, acute focal and diffuse glomerulonephritis and CNS symptoms like headache, diplopia and arthralgias and arthritis.

Direct immunofluorescence shows IgA, C3 C5 and fibrin within vessel walls. Histopathology shows two main cellular patterns of cutaneous necrotizing vasculitis which are leukocytoclastic form and lymphocytic form.

Leukocytoclastic form shows angiocentric segmental inflammation, swelling of endothelial cells, fibrinoid necrosis of blood vessels, cellular infiltration around and within dermal vessels composed largely of neutrophils showing fragmentation of nuclei and only a few lymphocytes, extravasation of erythrocytes and thrombosis of post capillary venules and hyalinisation of blood vessels in late stages.

Lymphocytic form shows swelling of endothelial cells, fibrin deposition extravasation of RBC and infiltrate composed largely of lymphocytes and macrophages.

Investigations include histopathology, immunofluorescence, test for rheumatoid factor, ANA, antiphospholipid antibodies, cryoglobulinemia, urine analysis to rule out proteinuria and haematuria.

Treatment

Various drugs like Corticosteroids, NSAIDS, Antimalarials, Colchicine 0.6 mg, Dapsone (50-100 mg/d), Potassium Iodide, Antihistaminics, Fibrinolytic agents, Aminocaproic acid (8-16 g/d), Immunosuppressive agents and monoclonal antibodies have been tried.

Dermatology Update

The ACR classification criteria for vasculitis

Temporal Arteritis Gaint cell (CGA)

1. Age >50 years at onset.
2. New type of headache.
3. Abnormal temporal artery on clinical examination (tenderness to palpation or decreased pulsation).
4. Elevated erythrocyte sedimentation rate.
5. Temporal artery biopsy showing vasculitis.

Three criteria classify CGA with sensitivity of 95.5% and specificity of 91.2%.

Takayasu's Arteritis (TA)

1. Age less than 40 years at onset.
2. Limb claudication.
3. Decreased brachial artery pulses.
4. BP >10 m Hg difference between two arms.
5. Bruits.
6. Arteriogram abnormal.

Three criteria classify TA with sensitivity of 90.5% and specificity of 97.8%.

Polyarteritis Nodosa (PAN)

1. Weight loss >4 kg.
2. Livedo reticularis.
3. Testicular pain or tenderness.
4. Myalgias, myopathy or tenderness.
5. Neuropathy.
6. Hypertension (diastolic BP >90 mm Hg).
7. Renal impairment (elevated BUN or creatinine).
8. Hepatitis B virus.
9. Abnormal arteriography.
10. Biopsy of artery showing PMN.

Three criteria classify PAN with sensitivity of 82.2% and specificity of 86.6%.

Wegner's Granulomatosis (WG)

1. Nasal or oral inflammation.

2. Chest X-ray showing nodules, infiltrates (fixed or cavities).
3. Microscopic hematuria or red cell casts in urine.
4. Granulomatous inflammation on biopsy (within vessel wall or perivascular).

Two criteria classify WG with sensitivity of 88.2% and specificity of 92.0%.

Churg-Strauss Syndrome (CSS)

1. Asthma.
2. Eosinophilia (>10%).
3. Neuropathy.
4. Pulmonary infiltrates (nonfixed).
5. Sinusitis.
6. Extravascular eosinophils on biopsy.

Four criteria classify CSS with sensitivity of 85% and specificity of 99.7%.

Hypersensitivity Vasculitis

1. Age > loyal onset.
2. Medications that may have precipitated event.
3. Palpable purpura.
4. Cutaneous eruption.
5. Positive biopsy results.

Three criteria classify HSV with sensitivity of 71.0% and specificity of 83.9%.

Henoch-Schönlein Purpura (HSP)

1. Palpable purpura.
2. Age at onset <20 years.
3. Bowel angina.
4. Vessel wall granulocytes on biopsy.

Two criteria classify HSP with sensitivity of 87% and specificity of 88%.

THE CHCC DEFINITIONS OF VASCULITIS

Large Vessel Vasculitis

Giant Cell (Temporal) Arteritis

Granulomatous arteritis of the aorta and its major branches, with a predilection for the extracranial branches of the carotid artery, often involves the temporal artery; usually occurs in patients older than 50 years and is often associated with polymyalgia rheumatica.

Takayasu Arteritis

Granulomatous inflammation of the aorta and its major branches, usually occurs in patients younger than 50 years.

Medium-sized Vessel Vasculitis

Polyarteritis Nodosa (Classic PAN)

Necrotizing inflammation of medium-sized or small arteries without glomerulonephritis or vasculitis inarterioles, capillaries, or venules.

Kawasaki Disease

Arteritis involving large, medium-sized or small arteries and associated with mucocutaneous lymph node syndrome; coronary arteries are often involved; aorta and veins may be involved; usually occurs in children.

Small Vessel Vasculitis

Wegner's Granulomatosis

Granulomatous inflammation involving the respiratory tract, and necrotizing vasculitis affecting small to medium-sized vessels (e.g. Capillaries, venules, arterioles and arteries); necrotizing glomerulonephritis is common.

Churg-Strauss Syndrome

Eosinophil-rich and granulomatous inflammation involving the respiratory tract, necrotizing vasculitis affecting small to medium-sized vessels, and associated with asthma and eosinophilia.

Microscopic Polyangitis

Necrotizing vasculitis, with few or no immune deposits, affecting small vessels (i.e., capillaries, venules or arterioles); necrotizing arteritis involving small and medium-sized arteries may be present; necrotizing glomerulonephritis is very common; pulmonary capillaritis often occurs.

Henoch-Schönlein Purpura

Vasculitis, with IgA-dominant immune deposits, affecting small vessels (i.e. Capillaries, venules, or arterioles); typically involves skin, gut, and glomeruli and is associated with arthralgias or arthritis.

Essential Cryoglobulinemic Vasculitis

Vasculitis, with cryoglobulin immune deposits, affecting small vessels (i.e. Capillaries, venules, or arterioles), and associated with cryoglobulins in serum; *skin and glomeruli are often involved.*

Cutaneous Leukocytoclastic Angitis

Isolated cutaneous leukocytoclastic angiitis without systemic vasculitis or glomerulonephritis.

MULTIPLE CHOICE QUESTIONS

1. **Palpable purpura is seen in following *except*:**
   A. ITP
   B. Henoch-Schönlein purpura
   C. Essential vascular cryoglobulinemia
   D. Scurvy
2. **Calciphylaxis is characterized by each of the following *except:***
   A. Vascular calcification
   B. Vasculitis
   C. Soft tissue necrosis
   D. Painful violaceous plaques that may ulcerate
3. **Severe abdominal pain may be a feature of:**
   A. Polyarteritis nodosa
   B. Henoch's purpura
   C. Erythema multiforme
   D. Erythema induratum

Chapter 13

Urticaria Angioedema

Urticaria: An eruption of transient erythematous or oedematous swelling of the dermis or subcutaneous tissue.

Angioedema or Angioneurotic oedema or Quinke's oedema or giant urticaria describe similar but larger swellings of the subcutaneous tissues.

Urticaria is due to a local increase in permeability of capillaries and small venules. Large number of substances present in the body are capable of mediating these changes of which histamine is best known others are prostaglandins, (D_2 I_2) **leukotrienes** ($B_4/C_4/D_4$), platelet activating factor, eosinophil and neutrophil chemotactic factors, kinins fibrin degradation products neuropeptides, serum factor etc.

Urticaria can be classified as follows:

1. Physical urticarias.
2. Cholinergic urticarias.
3. Hereditary angiodema.
4. Histamine releasing agents.
5. Allergic IgE mediated.
6. Allergic IgG mediated.
7. Idiopathic without significant aggravating factors.
8. Idiopathic with significant aggravating factors.
9. Rarer syndromes.

It can also be divided into:

1. Acute (of duration < 2 months).
2. Chronic (of duration > 2 months).

Also **Urticaria is often** classified as:

1. Allergic.
2. Non-allergic.

Provoking Factors

1. Physical agents → Heat, cold, pressure.
2. Drugs.
   - Foods and food additives.
   - Inhalants → Pollen, animal dander.
   - Infections → Respiratory, hepatitis, candida, helminthic.

Psychological Factors

General Medical Disorders: SLE, lymphoma, polycythemia, carcinoma, hypo and hyper thyroidism.

Types of physical urticaria and related disorders:

- Dermographism:
  - White.
  - Black.
- Delayed dermographism.
- Pressure urticaria.
- Solar urticaria.
- Cold urticaria.

- Heat urticaria.
- Cholinergic urticaria.
- Cholinergic pruritus.
- Aquagenic urticaria.
- Aquagenic pruritus.
- Vibratory angiodema.

Angioedema: Variant of urticaria where subcutaneous tissues, rather than dermis are mainly involved:

- Almost any part of body may be involved but most common sites are lips, eyelids and genitalia. Tongue and larynx may also be affected.
- Individual lesions may be single or multiple, may appear with dramatic suddenness, itching usually absent.
- Lesions last for a few hours or occasionally persist for 2 or 3 days.
- Treatment is same as for chronic urticaria.

Hereditary Angioedema

- Rare disorder → 1% of all cases of angioedema.
- Transmitted as autosomal dominant tract family history is usually found.
- Onset usually in early childhood but may be delayed into late adult like.
- Recurrent swellings of skin and mucous membranes often associated with nausea, vomiting, colic and urinary symptoms.
- Blood of these patients is deficient in natural inhibitor protein of first component of complement and of kallikrein and other enzymes.
- Response to conventional treatment is poor. Antihistamines and steroids are of little or no help.
- Attenuated androgen/anabolic drugs such as danazol and stanozolol—seem to stimulate production of the deficient inhibitor.
- Epsilon—amino caproic acid or tranexamine acid can control some cases.
- Replacement therapy with fresh frozen plasma can be helpful in severe acute prophylactically before surgery.

Acquired C_1 Esterase Inhibitor Deficiency

- Clinical picture is very similar but later in onset.
- May be associated with:
  - B cell lymphoma.
  - SLE.
  - An antibody directed against the inhibitor.
- *Treatment*—Danazol or steroids.

MULTIPLE CHOICE QUESTIONS

1. The biochemical study that is most accurate in distinguishing active from quiescent mast cell disease is determination of:

A. Serum histamine levels
B. Serum prostaglandin D_2 levels
C. Urinary histamine levels
D. Urinary methyl histamine levels

2. Sweet's syndrome has been reported to involve each of the following organs *except:*

A. Eye
B. Kidney
C. Lung
D. Uterus

3. Well's syndrome may precipitate by the following *except*:

A. Onchocerciasis
B. Fungal infections
C. Staphylococcal infection
D. Mumps

1 D 2 D 3 C

Chapter 14

Dermatologic Manifestations of Drugs

DERMATOLOGICAL EMERGENCIES

Dermatological emergencies are sudden, unexpected and undesirable contingency resulting secondary to the cutaneous pathology that needs a quick judgement and prompt action to prevent severe morbidity or death. These include: Erythroderma, erythema multiforme (Stevens Johnson syndrome and toxic epidermal necrolysis), drug reactions, urticaria and angioedema, vesiculobullous disorders like pemphigus and bullous pemphigoid.

Erythroderma (Syn. Exfoliative Dermatitis)

This term is applied to any inflammatory skin disease which affects more than 90% of the body surface. The condition presents as generalised erythema with scaling. The scales may be large, fine or bran-like. It is associated with burning, irritation, itching or a sensation of tightness. The disease occurs idiopathic and secondary to a number of causes that include eczemas (atopic, contact, seborrheic) in 40% cases, psoriasis (25%), drugs ingestion like arsenic, gold, mercury, rifampicin, INH, penicillins, barbiturates etc. (10%), other inflammatory skin disorders like lichenplanus, dermatophytosis, crusted scabies, pemphigus foliaceous, staphylococcal scalded skin syndrome, toxic shock syndrome, hereditary disorders like ichthyosiform erythroderma or malignancies like lymphomas, leukemia and carcinoma of the breasts bronchus, prostate etc. Males are affected two to three times, more frequently than females are usually over 45 years of age (excluding hereditary disorders and atopic dermatitis).

Erythroderma is associated with profound metabolic disturbances that may prove fatal despite skilled management, especially in elderly people with death rates varying from 18% to 64%. It may cause temperature dysregulation in the form of hypothermia or hyperthermia, excessive fluid loss, electrolyte imbalance, hypoalbuminemia, hypocalcemia and deficiency of iron, vitamin B_{12} and folic acid secondary to dermatogenic enteropathy and malabsorption, high output cardiac failure, hepatic and renal failure.

Management

This disease requires immediate hospitalization. Protein and electrolyte balance, body temperature, circulatory status require continuous surveillance. Adequate hydration should be maintained and cardiac, hepatic or renal failure must be promptly treated. Erythroderma secondary to drug reaction requires immediate withdrawal of the offending drug. Application of bland emolients prove to be very beneficial. Specific therapeutic modalities like methotrexate, azathioprine, cyclophosphamide, chlorambucil, cyclosporine and systemic corticosteroids are required according to the nature of the etiologic condition in severe persistent cases.

Erythema Multiforme (EM)

It is a syndrome with distinct clinical and histological features occurring as a reaction pattern to many different stimuli. It results from an immunological insult to the epidermal keratinocytes. Both delayed hypersensitivity and immune complex mechanisms have been proposed in its causation. An association with HLA B_{15} and DQW3 has also been reported.

This condition may occur secondary to various infections like viral herpes simplex, variola, vaccina, hepatitis B, milker's nodes, or, mumps, infectious mononucleosis, bacterial, chlamydial, rickettsial, fungal and protozoal infections. Other causes including immunologically mediated diseases like lupus erythematosus, polyarteritis nodosa, Wegener's granulomatosis, drug reaction to penicillins, sulphonamides, progesterone, barbiturates, rifampicin, dapsone etc., sarcoidosis, X-ray therapy or underlying carcinomas may initiate this disease.

Any age and both sexes may be involved. The disease presents as papular or simplex form with dull red, maculopapules with central purpura or cyanosis forming iris or target lesions. Classically the back of the hands, palms wrists, forearms, feet, elbows, knees and face are affected. In the vesiculobullous form the lesions present as erythematous plaques with central bulla and marginal ring of vesicles (Herpes iris of Bateman).

Stevens Johnson syndrome or EM major or severe bullous form of EM is a serious dermatological emergency with a suddenly onset of eruption. It is often preceded by a prodromal systemic illness of 1-13 days and numerous organs including the mouth, eyes, genitalia, anal mucosa, bronchi and lungs may be affected.

Besides the targetoid skin lesions, the mucous membrances show extensive bullae formation that rupture forming erosions covered by haemorrhagic crusts. Ophthalmologic complications like purulent conjunctivitis, corneal ulceration, anterior uveitis and panophthalmitis; renal involvement with haematuria, tubular necrosis or renal failure, polyarthritis and otitis media may occur.

This disease has a mortality of 5-15% mainly due to secondary infection, toxaemia or renal damage.

Toxic epidermal necrolysis is a very severe form of EM secondary to complete necrosis of the epidermis. The precise pathogenesis of the condition is not clear. However, a number of aetiological agents have been incriminated among which drugs like butazones, sulphonamides, phenolphthalein, phenytoin, pentazosine, ethambutol are the main aetiological agents.

The condition begins with fever and constitutional features followed by diffuse cutaneous erythema and tenderness. The Nikolsky sign is present over the erythematous skin and large areas of necrotic skin may be stripped off. Mucous membranes are extensively involved and healing may result in strictures and scarring with loss of hair and nails, corneal opacity and blindness. Mortality may occur in upto 25% patients.

Management

Treatment is mainly symptomatic and multidisciplinary. Good nursing care is of paramount importance. Topical therapy in the form of Condy's compresses ($KMnO_4$, 1,4000-1:16000) or Burrow's solution (Aluminium acetate solution) followed by topical and systemic antiobiotics is the mainstay of treatment. Antiviral therapy with acyclovir for erythema multiforme following overt herpes simplex infections tends to be disappointing. However long-term prophylactic use may be helpful.

The role of steroids is controversial. A high dose of systemic steroids in the early stages may hasten the subsidence of the lesions.

Cutaneous Drug Reactions

Drug reaction can be immunological and non-immunological:

- *Non-immunological drug* reactions can be due to:
  - – Direct releases of histamine from mast cells and basophils by opiates, polymyxin B, D-tubocurarine and radiocontrast media.
  - – Over dosage.
  - – Cumulative toxicity.
  - – Normal pharmacological effects that are not of primary therapeutic objective e.g. Alopecia following chemotherapy.
  - – Drug interactions.
  - – Metabolic changes → warfarin producing hypercoagulable state → warfarin necrosis.
  - – Exacerbation of preexisting dermatological disease e.g. Lithium can exacerbate acne, psoriasis and sub-corneal.
  - – Pustular dermatitis.
  - – Inherited enzyme or protein deficiencies.
  - – Intramuscular is the most likely parenteral way of eliciting drug sensitization, whereas intravenous is less likely. Oral route is least likely to produce sensitization.
  - – Cutaneous reactions are the most common adverse drug reactions e.g.→ pruritis, urticaria, angiodema, fixed drug eruptions, erythema multiformis, exfoliative dermatitis etc.
  - – Exanthema (maculopapular or morbilliform) drug eruptions are seen most commonly (46%) followed by urticaria and angioedema (26%) and FDE (10%).
  - – TEN is least common (1.3%) but most severe cut drug eruption.
  - – Amoxycillin and trimethoprim–sulfamethoxazole are most likely to produce cutaneous reactions.
  - – Chances of cut. adverse drug reaction to trimethoprim–sulfamethoxazole increases from 3% to 29-70% in patients with AIDS.
  - – In most cases TEN starts 1-3 weeks after starting the drug (Phenytoin requires 2-8 weeks) but if patient has had a similar eruption in the past–the time interval drops to < 48 hours.
  - – TEN is fatal in 25-70% of cases, secondary infection being the most common cause of death.
  - – Angioedema and anaphylaxis can result in quick death. They are IgE mediated reactions of the immediate hypersensitivity type.
  - – Most common class of drugs which can cause anaphylaxis → Beta-lactam antibiotics → mild pruritis, erythema, angiodema, asthma, circulatory collapse, laryngeal oedema and death.
  - – Treatment is required urgently with oxygen, IV hydrocortisone and adrenaline.
  - – The only useful specific lab tests are those dependent on their being specific immunoglobulin IgE directed to the particular drug. Penicillin is the only drug of importance that can be detected like this (by RAST→ radio-allergo adsorbent test).
  - – Intracutaneous prick and scratch tests may be helpful on rare occasions as with penicillin hypersensitivity.

DERMATOLOGIC MANIFESTATIONS OF DRUGS

ACNE

- Anabolic and androgenic steroids
- Bromides
- Glucocorticoids
- Iodides
- INH
- Oral contraceptives (OC)

- Troxidone
- Lithium

ALOPECIA
- Cytotoxics
- Ethionamide
- Heparin
- OC (withdrawal)

ECZEMA
- Captopril
- Cream and lotion
- Preservatives
- Lanolin
- Topical steroids
- Topical antihistamines
- Topical antimicrobials
- Topical local anaesthetics

ERYTHEMA MULTIFORME OR STEVENS-JOHNSON SYNDROME
- Barbiturate
- Chlorpropamide
- Codeine
- Ethosuximide
- Penicillins
- Phenylbutazone
- Phenytoin
- Salicylates
- Sulfonamides
- Sulfones
- Tetracycline
- Thiazides
- Carbamezapine.

ERYTHEMA NODOSUM
- OC (most common)
- Bromides
- Iodides
- Penicillins
- Sulfonamides

EXFOLIATIVE DERMATITIS
- Barbiturate
- Gold salts
- Penicillins
- Phenylbutazone
- Phenytoin
- Quinidine
- Sulfonamides

FIXED DRUG ERUPTIONS
- Barbiturate
- Captopril
- Phenolphthalein (most common)
- Phenylbutazone
- Quinine
- Betalactam antibiotics
- Tetracyclines
- Gold
- Salicylates
- Sulfonamides
- Dapsone
- Mefenemic acid

HYPERPIGMENTATION
- Busulphan
- Bleomycin
- Chloroquine
- Corticotropin
- Cyclophosphamide
- Gold salts
- Hypervitaminosis A
- OC
- Phenothiazines
- ACTH
- Zidovudine

LICHENOID ERUPTIONS
- Aminosalicylic acid
- Antimalarials
- Chlorpropamide
- Gold salts
- Methyldopa
- Phenothiazines
- Sulfonamides
- Thiazide diuretics
- Captopril
- Propanolol

PHOTODERMATITIS
- Captopril
- Chlordiazepoxide
- Frusemide
- Griseofulvin
- Nalidixic acid
- OC
- Phenothiazines
- Sulfonamides
- Sulfonylureas
- Demeclocycline (Tetracycline)
- Thiazides
- NSAID
- Amiodarone
- Quinidine
- Quinolones (Norfloxacin pefloxacin etc.)

PURPURA
- Aspirin
- Glucocorticoids

RASHES
- Allopurinol
- Ampicillin
- Barbiturate
- Indapamide
- Methyldopa
- Phenytoin

SKIN NECROSIS
- Warfarin

TOXIC EPIDERMAL NECROLYSIS (BULLOUS)
- Allopurinol
- Barbiturate
- Bromides
- Iodides
- Nalidixic acid
- Penicillins
- Phenylbutazone
- Phenolphthalein
- Phenytoin
- Sulfonamides
- Carbamezapine
- NSAIDS
- Gold salts

URTICARIA
- Aspirin
- Barbiturate
- Captopril
- Enalapril
- Penicillins
- Sulfonamides
- Blood products

PSEUDOPORPHYRIA LIKE RASH
- Naproxen
- Frusemide
- Tetracycline
- Nalidixic acid
- Sulfonamides
- Dapsone
- Pyridoxine

LUPUS ERYTHEMATOUS LIKE RASHES
- Penicillamine
- Hydralazine
- Hydantoins
- Procainamide
- INH
- Chlorpromazine
- Methyldopa
- Quinidine

URTICARIA
- Penicillins
- Aspirin
- Blood products

SERUM SICKNESS LIKE DRUG RASHES
- Betalactam antibiotics
- Sulfonamides
- Thiouracil
- Cholecystographic lyes
- Hydantoin

ANGIOEDEMA
- Captopril
- Enalapril
- Lisenopril

Drugs producing changes in skin pigmentation:

Slate gray	–	Chloroquine Hydroxychloroquine Minocycline Phenothiazines
Slate blue	–	Amiodarone
Blue gray	–	Gold (chrysoderma)
Yellow	–	Beta carotene Quinacrine
Red	–	Clofazimine
Brown (hyper-pigmentation)	–	ACTH Bleomycin OC Zidovudine Busulfan Hypervitaminosis A Phenothiazines Cyclophosphamide

MULTIPLE CHOICE QUESTIONS

1. **Acneiform eruptions are seen with all *except*:**
   A. Anabatic steroids
   B. Bromides and iodides
   C. INH
   D. OCPs
   E. Rifampicin

2. **Drugs causing erythema multiform are all *except*:**
   A. Penicillin
   B. Sulfonamides
   C. Prenothiazines
   D. Digoxin

3. **State like discoloration of the skin is caused by all these drugs *except*:**
   A. Chlorpromazine
   B. Minocycline
   C. Amiodarone
   D. Thiaceta zone

4. **Most common cause of "fixed" drug eruption:**
   A. Barbiturates
   B. Sulphonamides
   C. Phenolpththalein
   D. Salicylates

5. **Lichenoid eruptions are caused by:**
   A. Aminosalicylic acid
   B. Gold salts
   C. Phenothiazines
   D. Antimalarials
   E. All of the above

6. **Photodermatitis is caused by:**
   A. Frusemide
   B. Nalidixic acid
   C. Griseofulvin
   D. Phenothiazines
   E. All of the above

7. **Photo-onycholysis is seen as an adverse effect of:**
   A. Phenytoin
   B. Chlorpromazine
   C. Chloramphenicol
   D. Demeclocycline

8. **Urticaria and angioedema are caused due to release of:**
   A. Serotonin
   B. Histamine
   C. Prostaglandin
   D. Adrenalin

9. **Which of the following investigations is used in detecting drug eruptions?**
   A. RAST
   B. Immunofluorescent antibody test
   C. Histamine test
   D. Skin patch testing

10. **Which of the following drugs cause hypermelanosis?**
   A. Busulfan
   B. Bleomycin
   C. Cyclophosphamide
   D. Adriamycin
   E. All of the above

11. **The most frequent side-effect of isotretinoin is:**
   A. Chest pain
   B. Cheilitis
   C. Arthralgia
   D. Dizziness

1 E 2 D 3 C 4 C 5 E 6 E 7 D 8 B 9 A 10 E 11 B

12. Albinism is a known adverse effect of:
A. Chloroquine
B. Procaine
C. Digitalis
D. Phenacetin

13. Black hairy tongue is caused by:
A. Pentamidine
B. Verapamil
C. Quinine
D. Tetracycline

14. Following drugs cause photosensitization *except*:
A. Tetracycline
B. Phenothiazine
C. Amiodarone
D. Digoxin

15. Which of the following drug is associated with urticaria?
A. Penicillin
B. Opioids
C. Aspirin
D. All of the above

16. Drug of choice in acute severe angioedema is:
A. Tefenadine
B. Promethazine
C. Hydrocortisone
D. Cimetidine

17. Which of the following investigations is used in detecting drug eruptions?
A. RAST
B. Immunofluorescent antibody test
C. Histamine test
D. Skin patch testing

18. Pseudoporphyria like rash is seen as a side effect of:
A. Frusemide
B. Phenytoin
C. Digoxin
D. Verapamil

19. Acneiform drug eruptions can be caused by all *except*:
A. Corticosteroids
B. Iodides
C. INH
D. Oral contraceptives
E. Phenytoin

20. Fixed drug eruptions are commonly caused by all *except*:
A. Barbiturates
B. Sulfonamides
C. Salicylates
D. Penicillins

21. Photodermatitis is caused by:
A. Frusemide
B. Nalidixic acid
C. Griseofulvin
D. Phenothiazines
E. All of the above

22. Secondary ichthyosis of skin is produced by all *except*:
A. Nicotinic acid
B. Stilboesterol
C. Phenobarbitone
D. Butyrophenones

23. Most common complication of systemic therapy retinoid is:
A. Dry mouth and skin
B. Headache
C. Alopecia
D. Bone pain

24. Most frequent adverse reaction to dapsone is:
A. Haemolysis
B. Anaphylaxis
C. Fixed drug eruption
D. Agranulocytosis

12 A 13 D 14 D 15 D 16 C 17 A 18 A 19 E 20 D 21 E 22 C
23 A 24 A

25. Nephrotoxicity is a prominent side effect of:
- A. Griseofulvin
- B. Amphotericin-B
- C. Hamycin
- D. Clotrimazole

26. Antileprosy drug contraindicated in G-6-P-D deficiency:
- A. Rifampicin
- B. Clofazimine
- C. Dapsone
- D. None of the above

27. Which of the following drugs cause melanosus?
- A. Busulfan
- B. Bleomycin
- C. Cyclophosphamide
- D. Adriamycin
- E. All of the above

28. Causes of non-melanin skin pigmentation are all *except*:
- A. Ochronosis
- B. Carotinaemia
- C. Haemosiderosis
- D. Argyria

29. Placentrex lotion is used in the therapy of:
- A. Psoriasis
- B. Alopecia areata
- C. Vitiligo
- D. Pemphigus

30. Riehl's melanosis is most common on:
- A. Upper arm
- B. Legs
- C. Chest
- D. Face

31. Minoxidil is safe for use in .... years age group:
- A. 3-45
- B. 12-60
- C. 18-65
- D. 18-45

32. Miconazole has the following effect:
- A. Antifungal
- B. Antibacterial
- C. Antiviral
- D. All of the above

33. Topical steroids may be used in the following *except*:
- A. Lichen rosacea
- B. Acne rosacea
- C. Seborrhoeic dermatitis
- D. Alopecia areata

34. Peripheral neuritis may be a side-effect of:
- A. Griseofulvin
- B. Fluconazole
- C. Ketoconazole
- D. Miconazole

35. Drug most useful in acne venenata is:
- A. Ciclopirox olamine
- B. Tretinoin
- C. Benzoyl peroxide
- D. Amlodepine

36. True about topical steroid use in children is all *except*:
- A. Potent steroid use can lead to growth retardation
- B. Limit use in children to 5 days
- C. Use mild or moderately potent steroids only
- D. Withdraw suddenly if there is no improvement

25 B 26 C 27 E 28 D 29 C 30 D 31 C 32 A 33 B 34 A 35 B 36 D

Chapter 15

Alopecia's Physiology

2-6 years

Anagen ——→ Catagen

| |

Hair shedding ←—— Telogen100 days

Hair Cycle

90% of our terminal hairs are at anagen phase which is the growing phase. It lasts for 2-6 years. The scalp hair on average grows at the rate of 0.37 mm per day.

Catagen is a transient period. Hair matrix cells stop dividing. As a result, there is no hair growth.

Less than 10% of our hairs should be in telogen phase which lasts for 100 days (about 3 months). Since on average, each person has about 100,000 hairs. Therefore, less than 10,000 should be in telogen phase and on each day less *than 100 hairs fall off physiologically.*

Physiological hair loss is defined as the loss of < 100 hair/day. Alopecia is the term used to denote loss of hair localized to the scalp. Pathological hair loss can be congenital or acquired. Depending on the morphology, pathological hair loss can be scarring or non-scarring.

Scarring Alopecia

- Injury.
- Infections like favus, kerion, furunculosis.
- Autoimmune disorders (lichen planus, lupus erythematosus, morphoea).
- Radio-dermatitis.

Scarring alopecia: Suggested therapies

Lichen planopilaris	Systemic steroids + topical minoxidil Azathioprine + systemic steroids + topical minoxidil
Fibrosing alopecia in a pattern distribution	Finasteride + systemic steroids
OLE	Hydroxychloroquine Hydroxychloroquine + systemic steroids
Folliculitis decalvans	Rifampicin + clindamycin Tetracyclines Clarithromycin
KFSD	Retinoids Dapsone Tetracyclines
Localized scleroderma	Oral calcitriol Penicillin

Non Scarring Alopecia

Patchy alopecia-androgenetic alopecia, alopecia areata, trichotillomania or various infections).

Diffuse alopecia—telogen effluvium or drug induced alopecia or secondary to systemic diseases such as lupus erythematosus, occult malignancies.

Male Pattern Baldness (Androgenetic Alopecia)

This is a misnomer, and can lead to missed diagnosis in a female. The essential feature is the replacement of terminal hair by vellus hair which are short and unpigmented. The process begins after puberty with a uniform fronto-temporal recession and later involving the vertex as well.

This is believed to be due to androgenic stimulation of the hair follicles. However, there is no evidence of excess androgens and the follicles overreact to normal levels of androgens due to genetic and ageing factors.

Treatment

Medical—Topical minoxidil, oral antiandrogens like finasteride, flutamide, oral contraceptives.

Surgical—Hair grafting.

Telogen effluvium: It represents excess shedding of hair (>100/day) which are in resting (telogen) phase of hair cycle.

Causes: Several factors such as surgery, anaemia, Vitamin B_{12} deficiency, folic acid, deficiency, parturition, rapid weight loss, acute febrile illness, drugs (anticoagulants, β-blockers) and endocrinal problem (hypo-hyperthyroidism, hyperpituitarism are incriminated.

Hair loss usually occurs 2-3 months after the causative agent, continues for 3-6 months but always terminates in recovery.

Increase in the proportion of resting telogen hair follicles. Diffuse thinning of hair with increase shedding of hair is the striking features. It is a soft limiting condition and the treatment consists of assurance and care of underlying cause. In chronic cases, 2% minoxidil solution can be used topically.

Alopecia Areata

It is an autoimmune disorder characterised by patchy or confluent hair loss on the scalp and /or body.

Alopecia totalis refers to total loss of scalp hair while alopecia universalis represents total loss of body and scalp hair. Ophiasis refers to the extension of alopecia along scalp margin. The underlying skin appears normal in alopecia areata. The anagen phase is abruptly terminated prematurely and the affected hair move into telogen phase with resultant patchy hair loss. ***Exclamation point hair,*** the pathognomic signs are present at the periphery of hair loss.

Alopecia areata is often associated with other auto immune disorders like thyroiditis, pernicious anaemia, vitiligo etc.

Treatment: It is a self-limiting disorder. The patient needs assurance and treatment includes topical irritants, corticosteroids, 2% minoxidil lotion. Refractory cases may need systemic steroids or other immunosuppressants (cyclosporin) or contact sensitization with DCP.

Traumatic alopecia is applied to alopecia induced by physical trauma. Alopecia resulting from the deliberate, at times unconscious efforts of the patients who are under tension or psychologically disturbed is called ***trichotillomania.*** It is twice as more common in females than in males and peak incidence is 11-17 years in females and 2-6 years in males. The patient twists hair around fingers and pulls it resulting in the breakage of hair. The sites most frequently involved are the frontal and parietal regions. This results in illdefined patch with twisted hair broken at various distances from clinically normal scalp. Most characteristically, the plucked area covers the entire scalp apart from the margin. This is called Tonsure alopecia or Orentriech sign.

Treatment includes psychological and behavioural therapy.

MULTIPLE CHOICE QUESTIONS

1. Pohl-Pinkus lines on hairs are:
A. Analogus to Beau's lines on nails
B. Same as Langer's line of cleavage
C. Embryonic marker of prematurity
D. None of the above

2. The optimum duration of treatment for an effective response with topical minoxidil in male-type alopecia is:
A. 2-4 weeks B. 2-3 months
C. 3-6 months D. 6-12 months

3. Folliculitis decalvans is more common on:
A. Scalp B. Face
C. Extremities D. Groin

4. Features which carry a bad prognosis in alopecia areata include:
A. Peripheral scalp involvement
B. Extensive initial involvement
C. Both of the above
D. None of the above

5. Sudden "overnight" graying of hair is apparently due to:
A. Drying of hair with development of hair space
B. Loss of pigmented hair, leaving the gray
C. Chemical dissolution of the melanin
D. All of the above
E. None of the above

6. Exclamation marks hair are seen in:
A. Cicatricial alopecia
B. Alopecia areata
C. Syphilitic alopecia
D. Alopecia totalis

7. Aetiology of alopecia acreata is:
A. Androgenetic stimulation
B. Infective
C. Autoimmune
D. Traumatic

8. The recommended concentration of minoxidil for topical application is:
A. < 1%
B. 1-2%
C. 2-5%
D. 5-10%

9. The patients with alopecia areata have a greater incidence of:
A. Thyroid disease
B. Vitiligo
C. Onychodystrophies
D. All of the above
E. None of the above

10. Features which carry a bad prognosis in alopecia areata include:
A. Peripheral scalp involvement
B. Extensive initial involvement
C. Both of the above
D. None of the above

11. Common female baldness (androgen-mediated) shows:
A. Fronto-parietal recession
B. Diffuse hair loss
C. Eventual complete baldness
D. None of the above

1 A 2 D 3 A 4 B 5 B 6 B 7 C 8 C 9 D 10 C 11 B

12. Therapy of alopecia areata is generally unsatisfactory but is probably best treated with:

A. Radiation
B. Sulfonamide cream
C. Systemic steroids
D. Local injection of triamcinolone acetonide suspension

13. Cicatrical alopecia is usually caused by all of the following *except:*

A. Kerion
B. Folliculitis decalvans
C. Graham-Little syndrome
D. Pseudopelade

12 D 13 A

Chapter 16

Leprosy

- Also called **Hansen's disease.** Caused by Mycobacterium leprae.
- M. leprae was discovered by **Gerhard Armauer Hansen** in 1873 at Norway. It was the first bacillus to be associated with human disease.
- M. leprae was cultured in foot pad of mice by **Shephard** in 1960.
- 70 % of world load is in India.
- India = majority are PB.
- Main mode of exit is **nasal mucosa** of untreated cases. Although mode of transmission is still uncertain it seems most likely that M. leprae are transmitted via naso-respiratory route.
- Dangers of infection is from only open cases, who are not taking treatment.
- Characteristics virulence factor of M. leprae is **phenolic glycolipid I,** a prominent surface lipid, specific of this bacillus.
- Generation time is **12 days; Incubation period is 2-7 years** (average 3-5 years).
- **Common sites** of involvement are: Skin, peripheral nerve but leprosy can involve every organ except CNS and lungs.
- Transplacental transmission does not occur commonly.
- Target organ of M. leprae is **Schwan cells** of peripheral nerves.
- Risk of transmission of leprosy from a marriage partner is only 5% (Conjugal leprosy).
- Risk of children acquiring infection from infected adults in the family is 60%.
- In high resistance persons, **tuberculoid leprosy** occurs.
- In low resistance persons, **lepromatous leprosy** occurs.
- In India, tuberculoid leprosy is **more common** than lepromatous leprosy.
- Earliest sensation lost is **thermal sensation** (cold before hot).
- Cranial nerves commonly involved are trigeminal and facial.
- Most common nerve to be involved is ulnar nerve.
- **Cardinal signs of leprosy are:**
  - i. Area of absent or decreased sensation.
  - ii. Thickened and/or tender nerves.
  - iii. Demonstration of M. leprae in the skin.

Any Two (NLEP)

- **Classification of leprosy:**

  PB—1-5 skin lesions.

  MB— > 5 lesions.

  Polyneuritic > 1–MB.

  SSL—single skin lesions—a lesion with sensory loss but no nerve enlargement or infiltration.

Based on Clinical, Bacteriological, Immunological and Histological Findings

- Two **stable** polar types:
  - i. Lepromatous (LL).
  - ii. Tuberculoid (TT).

- Two **unstable** polar types:
  - i. Indeterminate and (I).
  - ii. Borderline (B).
- **Borderline** types are of 3 types:
  - i. Borderline tuberculoid (BT).
  - ii. Mid borderline (MB).
  - iii. Borderline lepromatous (BL).

INDETERMINATE LEPROSY

- Patient is usually a child.
- One or more hypopigmented faintly **macules** erythematous.
- Outer edges → ill defined to well defined.
- More likely to be present on covered areas.
- Anaesthesia slight or absent.
- Slit smear for AFB → negative—but occasional AFB may be seen within a cut. Nerve on Biopsy.
- Sometimes thickened nerve palpable.
- **Usually heals spontaneously; about 30% progress to determinate types → more often towards L.L. pole.**

NEURAL LEPROSY

- Form of leprosy with one or more enlarged nerves but no skin lesions.
- Nerve biopsy necessary for diagnosis.
- MB>1nerve.
- Lepromin test of great value in classification:
  → strongly + in TT.
  → weakly + in BT.
  → negative in BB, BL, LL.
- Treatment → MDT; steroids if thickened nerves are painful + tender.

LUCIO LEPROSY

- Described in Mexico.
- Diffuse non-nodular.

	TT	*BT*	*BB*	*BL*	*LL*
Cutaneous lesion	Hypopig/erythematous macules/ plaques well defined, regular dry, scaly **usually complete loss of sweating.** Partial/complete loss of hair. Sensations lost. Number usually < 3 Thickened or tender or both, nerves feeding the patch	Hypopig/erythematous macules/ plaques well defined, irregular margins dry, scaly, **satellite lesions.** Impaired/complete loss of sweating. Partial/complete loss of hair. Sensations impaired. Number usually <10 Nerves supplying patches are thickened/tender or both	Lesions show morphology of tuberculoid as well as lepromatous. Lesions are bilateral but asymmetrical. Number is numerous but countable. Sensations ↓ with ↓ hair growth. Nerves- thickened/tender or both	Variable morphology - Tuberculoid - Lepromatous Shiny, bilateral, tending to be symmetrical. Numerous and uncountable. Sensations slightly ↓, hair slightly ↓. Nerves- thickened/tender or both	Small, shiny, bilaterally, symmetrical, hypopig/erythematous macules, plaque papules nodules. Margins ill defined usually no impairment of sweating. Numerous and uncountable. Multiple nerves thickened. Loss of eyebrows and eyelashes in filtrated sys. involvement
Immunology (lepromin)	Strongly positive (+++)	Weakly positive (+ or ++)	Negative (–)	Negative (–)	Negative (–)
Histopath	Compact granuloma (tuberculoid) hugging or eroding epidermis. Cutaneous nerves → destroyed or swollen/caseation	Tuberculoid granuloma less compact than TT. Subepid, grenz-zone appears. Nerves → cellular infiltrate	Diffuse epitheloid cell granuloma Grenz zone + nerves → infiltrated	Granuloma composed of macrophages + lymphocytes. Grenz zone + Nerves Nerves infiltrated	Thinned epider. Diffuse lepromatous foamy macrophages few. Lymphocytes + plasma cells. Grenz zone cut nerves are preserved
Bacteriology (slit smear)	NO AFB seen	Nil or scanty AFB	Moderate no.	Many	Very many (plus globulin)

- Shiny thickened skin, loss of body and facial hair, puffy hands, chronic oedema and ulceration of legs.
- Widespread sensory loss.
- Eyes → shiny, thickened upper eyelids → sleepy look.
- Ulceration of nasal mucosa → epistaxis.
- Laryngeal involvement → hoarse voice.
- Develop peculiar form of lepra reaction → LUCIO PHENOMENON.

HISTOID LEPROSY—VARIANT OF LL

- Term introduced by Wade.
- Type of lepromatous leprosy but with better C.M.I.
- Usually seen in patients whose disease is relapsing due to:
  - i. Stoppage of treatment.
  - ii. Drug resistance.
- Skin lesions → firm, erythematous, round to oval, shiny, succulent nodules.
- AFB seen of slit smear → longer, lying singly or in parallel bundles.
- Treatment—MB-MDT.

PREGNANCY AND LEPROSY

- Worsening of disease especially in IIIrd trimester since ↓ CMI.
- **Type 1 reaction especially during first 6 months postpartum → due to regaining of C.M.I.**
- **Type 2 reaction** → esp. in IIIrd trimester and first 6 months of lactation → since physical stress and return to normal of plasma ACTH + cortisol levels.
- Almost **50% suffer deterioration of nerve function.**
- Babies born to mothers with leprosy weighed less and grew more slowly.
- Rifampicin, Dapsone and Elofazimine, all 3 drugs are considered safe in pregnancy.

Reaction in Leprosy

Reactions are acute episodes of hypersensitivity reactions due to fluctuations in the immune status of a leprosy patient. There are three types of reactions; type 1 reaction, type 2 reaction and Lucio phenomenon.

Type 1 lepra reaction (reversal reaction):

- It is type IV hypersensitivity reaction (Coombs and Gell type).
- Seen in borderline spectrum (BT, BB, BL).
- May manifest in the skin or nerve lesions of leprosy.
- Erythema, edema and hyperalgesia of existing skin lesions occurs. Occurrence of new lesions—downgrading.
- Rarely ulcerations of skin lesions.
- Excruciatingly tender and thickened nerves with sensory or motor deficit.
- Patient can develop nerve palsies and in severe reactions oedema of the hands and feet (No constitutional symptoms usually seen).
- Most important aspect of type 1 lepra reaction is not the skin lesions but the condition of peripheral nerves.
- Mild reaction can be managed with analgesics.
- Severe reaction and neuritis needs oral steroids, commonly prednisolone is used in the dose of 30 to 40 mg per day.

Type 2 lepra reaction:

- It is a type III or immune complex mediated lepra reaction.
- Occurs in lepromatous spectrum (Most commonly in LL, occasionally in BL).
- Triggered by infection, vaccination, drugs and stress.
- Characterized by tender, erythematous, evanescent nodules called as erythema nodosum leprosum (ENL).

- ENL occurs over the face and extensors.
- ENL does not occur in legs in contrast to erythema nodosum which occurs in legs.
- Constitutional symptoms such as fever, arthralgia, anorexia and myalgia occur.
- May have systemic involvement in the form of conjunctivits, keratitis, iritis, iridocyclitis, orchitis, hepatomegaly and lymphadenopathy.
- Treatment is with corticosteroids and thalidomide.

Systemic

- Most common cause of death in lepromatous leprosy is **Renal failure.**
- Type of anaemia seen in leprosy is **Dimorphic** anaemia.
- Cause of blindness in lepromatous variety is due to **iridiocyclitis.**
- Cause of blindness in tuberculoid variety is exposure **keratitis** due to lagophthalmos.
- Type I lepra reaction is seen in **borderline leprosy,** due to **cell mediated immunity** (Type IV hypersensitivity).
- Type II lepra reaction is seen in **lepromatous** and **borderline lepromatous** type. It is a type of **antigen antibody reaction** (Type III hypersensitivity).
- Skin lesion in type II reactions are **tender**, red nodules plaque, distributed bilaterally **symmetrically**, mainly on face, arm and thigh. These lesions are evanescent.
- Erythema Nodosum Leprosum (ENL) is found in type II reaction.
- Lepromin test has no role in diagnosis, rather it has got importance in **prognosis** and classification of leprosy into various subtypes.

Treatment

- According to WHO, **a paucibacilliary cases** are the cases where, bacteriological index is zero.
- **Rifampicin** is the most rapidly acting bactericidal drug against M. leprae. Half life of Rifampicin is 4-5 hours.
- Side Effects of Rifampicin are:
  - Red discolouration of urine.
  - Abdominal pain, gastrointestinal symptoms.
  - Skin rash.
  - Thrombocytopenia.
  - Flu like syndrome (due to intermittent administration).
  - Serious side-effects (uncommon) include → hepatitis, psychosis, thrombocytopenia, osteomalacia, hypersensitivity reactions like Stevens Johnson syndrome, porphyria cutanea tarda and pemphigus vulgaris.
  - Dapsone was discovered by **Cochrane** in 1941.
  - Dose of Dapsone is 1-2 mg/kg. It is a **bacteriostatic** drug.
  - Half life of Dapsone is 24 hours.
  - Most frequent adverse effect of Dapsone is Hemolysis (individuals deficient in G6PD are more prone).
- Other side effects of Dapsone are:
  - Methaemoglobinaemia.
  - Agranulocytosis mild thrombocytopenia.
  - Psychosis.
  - Hepatitis.
  - Skin Rash (exanthematous), exfoliative dermatitis, toxic epidermal necrolysis, Stevens Johnson syndrome, Fixed Drug eruptions.
  - Polyneuropathy.
  - Insomnia, Irritability.
  - Dapsone syndrome (DDS Syndrome).
- Minimum lethal dose of Dapsone in mice is 0.30 mg/dl.
- **Secondary resistance to Dapsone is most common in Lepromatous patients, Resistance develops as a result of multi step mutation.**

- **Drug of choice in type I lepra reaction is corticosteroid. Type I reaction does not respond to thalidomide.**
- **Drug of choice in type II lepra is thalidomide. Other drugs used are corticosteroid and clofazamine.**
- Antileprosy drugs should not be stopped during reaction phase or during pregnancy.
- Nerve abscess needs incision and drainage.
- Clofazimine is iminophenazine dye. It has dual effect.
- Clofazimine is bacteriostatic against M leprae and anti-inflammatory against lepra reaction.
- Dose of clofazimine is 300-350 mg/wk (50 mg daily).
- The dose in lepra reaction is 300 mg/daily.
- Side effects are:

  Skin and conjunctiva pigmentation (red brown discoloration), red colouration of urine, stools, sputum, sweat, tears.
- Icthysosis particularly over forearms and legs.
- GI disturbances like diarrhea.

Treatment (Medical)

Multi-drug therapy for Multi-bacillary (MB) leprosy

	RFP	*Dapsone*	*CLF*
Adult			
50-70 kg	600 mg/m	100 mg/d	50 mg/d and 300 mg/m
Child			
10-14 years (10-14) *	450 mg/m	50 mg/d	50 mg/d and 150 mg/m
Less than 10 (6-9) *	300 mg/m	25 mg/d	50 mg twice/w and 100 mg/m

Multi-drug therapy for pauci-bacillary (PB) leprosy

	PFP	*Dapsone*
Adult		
50-70 kg	600 mg/m	100 mg/d
Child		
10-14 years (0-5)*	450 mg/m	50 mg/d
Less than 10 (6-14)*	300 mg/m	25 mg/d

Multi-drug Therapy for Single Lesion Pauci-bacillary (SLPB) Leprosy

(Not recommended for pregnant women and children less than 5 years old)

	PFP	*OFLX*	*MINO*
Adult			
50-70 kg	600 mg	400 mg	100 mg
Child			
5-14 years +	300 mg	200 mg	50 mg

Drugs used in MDT

RFP	Bactericidal
Dapsone	Bacteriostatic, weakly bactericidal
CLF	Slow bactericidal
OFLX	Bactericidal
MINO	Bacteriostatic
SPFX	Bactericidal
CAM	Bacteriostatic, weakly bactericidal

Accompanied-MDT(A-MDT)—Give the full course on the first visit.

Uniform MDT (U–MDT)—6 month to all patients.

NEWER DRUGS IN LEPROSY

1. Quinolones—Perfloxacin, ofloxacin, ciprofloxacin, sparfloxacin.
2. Tetracyclines—Minocycline.
3. Macrolides—Clarithromycin, Roxithromycin.
4. Dapsone analogs.
5. Clofazimine derivatives.
6. Ansamycins—Rifamycin, Rifapentine, Rifabutine.
7. Aminoglycosides—Streptomysin.
8. Cephalosporins—Cefoxitin,Cephaloridin.
9. Beta lactams.
10. DiHydro folate reductase inhibitors—Brodimoprim, Pyrimethamine.
11. Tyrosine inhibitors—Deoxyfructoserotonin.
12. Pyrazinamide.
13. MRRI mycobacterium ribonucleotide reductase inhibitors.
14. Amoxycillin + Clavulanic acid.
15. Fucidic acid.

LEPROSY

LEPROSY: Latest data: India.

2006 March Prevalence → 0.9/10000.

On treatment → 5.1 lakhs.

Maximum prevalence → Bihar, Orissa, West Bengal, Tamilnadu, UP.

ROM therapy.

Single dose therapy for single lesion of leprosy consisting of:

Rifampicin → 600 mg

Ofloxacin → 400 mg

Minocycline → 100 mg

Vaccines for Leprosy: To be used for:

a. Immunoprophylaxis.

b. Immunotherapy.

FIRST GENERATION VACCINES

BCG vaccine.

Killed M leprae (armadillo).

Killed M leprae+live BCG (CONVIT).

Killed cross reacting M leprae and chemically modified M leprae (which are cultivable).

a. M welchii (Talwars).

b. ICRC bacillus vaccine (DEO's).

c. M vaccae (Stanfords).

d. M leprae-DCC (Mahadevans).

e. Vaccine from M habana (Singhs).

SECOND GENERATION VACCINES

70KD;65KD;31KD;18KD;10KD vaccines.

THIRD GENERATION VACCINES

Recombinant DNA vaccines.

MULTIPLE CHOICE QUESTIONS

1. **A 45-year-old male had multiple hypo-aesthetic mildly erythematous large plaques with elevated margins on trunk and extremities. His ulnar and lateral popliteal nerves on both sides were enlarged. The most probable diagnosis is:**
   A. Lepromatous leprosy
   B. Borderline leprosy
   C. Borderline tuberculoid leprosy
   D. Borderline lepromatous leprosy
2. **A 40-year-old tailor complains of pain, numbness and weakness of the right hand for the last three months. On examination, there is hypoasthesia and atrophy of thenar eminence. Which one of the following nerves is likely to be involved?**
   A. Ulnar
   B. Radial
   C. Axillary
   D. Median
3. **In Ridley Jopling classification of leprosy which of the following term is not used?**
   A. Lepromatous leprosy
   B. Borderline leprosy
   C. Indeterminate leprosy
   D. Histoid leprosy
4. **Treatment of choice for single lesion of leprosy (WHO):**
   A. ROM therapy
   B. 6 months of PB-MDT
   C. Immunotherapy
   D. No treatment required → just observe
5. **Inverted saucer appearance in leprosy is seen in:**
   A. Borderline borderline
   B. Tuberculoid
   C. Lepromatous
   D. Borderline tuberculoid
6. **All of the following statements about leprosy are true *except*:**
   A. Multibacillary leprosy is diagnosed when there are more than 5 skin patches
   B. New case detection rate is an indicator for incidence of leprosy
   C. A defaulter is defined as a patient who has not taken treatment for 6 months or more
   D. The target for elimination of leprosy is to reduce the prevalence to less than 1 per 10,000 population
7. **All of the following are the mode of transmission of leprosy *except:***
   A. Breast milk
   B. Insect bite
   C. Transplacental spread
   D. Droplet infection
8. **Type II Lepra reaction is .... type hypersensitivity (Coomb–Gel) reaction:**
   A. I
   B. II
   C. III
   D. IV

1 B 2 D 3 C,D 4 A 5 A 6 C 7 C 8 C

9. **Swiss cheese pattern of skin lesions are seen in:**
   A. BB Hansens
   B. BT Hansens
   C. LL Hansens
   D. TT Hansens

10. **Which of the following is not effective in erythema nodosum leprosum?**
    A. NSAIDS
    B. Antimalarials
    C. Antimonials
    D. High doses of dapsone

9 A 10 D

Chapter 17

Skin Tumours

Derivation of benign skin tumours

Part of skin	*Benign skin tumour*
• Melanocytes	Junctional melanocytic naevus, compound melanocytic naevus, intradermal melanocytic naevus
• Epidermal keratinocytes	Basal cell papilloma (seborrhoeic keratosisi), solar keratosis
• Hair follicles	Epidermoid cyst (also termed 'pilar cyst')
• Fibroblasts in dermis	Dermatofibroma
• Blood vessels	Spider naevi, Campbell de Morgan spots, pyogenic granuloma

BASAL CELL CARCINOMA

BCC is the most common tumor in humans. The diagnosis of BCC is seldom made in patients younger than age 40 and has been more common in men.

Dermatologic conditions that predispose a patient to the development of BCC include Jadassohn's sebaceous naevus, linear epidermal naevus, albinism, xeroderma pigmentosum (UV-induced DNA dimer excision-repair defect), Rasmussen's syndrome, Rombo syndrome, Bazex's syndrome, and basal cell naevus syndrome (patched gene human homologue defect).

BCC distribution parallels that of pilosebaceous follicles and sun-exposed skin, both greatest on the head and neck. BCC may appear on nonfollicular skin but almost never arises from the oral, anal or vaginal mucosa.

Clinical Characteristics and Course

The concept of 'low-risk' and 'high-risk' BCC has been described in order to allow the clinician to choose the most appropriate form of treatment. Factors determining these risk factors are: tumour size, type and site, definition of tumour margins, histological type and growth pattern, recurrent tumours and finally immunocompromised patients.

Primary BCC

BCC grows slowly, is painless and frequently ignored by the patient. If metastases are rare, local invasion could be destructive when tumours are neglected. In such cases, the tumour may infiltrate in depth through the different tissue layers into the cranial cavity or along the embryological fusion planes, provoking important morbidity or eventually a fatal outcome.

Diagnosis of the clinical variants is of great importance as the choice of treatment modality depends on the clinical type of the BCC.

Special attention should be paid to the basosquamous and metatypical type of BCC. Initially,

Main characteristics of clinical BCC subtypes

Clinical subtypes	*Localization*	*Growth*	*Lesion*	*Colour*	*Surface*
Solid nodular	Face	Slow	Nodule	Skin translucent	Telangiectasia
Rodent ulcer	Face	Faster	Central ulcer coiled border	Translucent necrotic, red	Telangiectasia
Pigmented	Face	Slow	Nodule	Browth	Telangiectasia
Adenocystic	Face	Slow	Lobulated cyst + rolled edge	Erythmatous/ +squamous Translucent	Telangiectasia
Superficial	Trunk Limbs	Slow	Plaque pearly border	Red scaly	Well defined
Morphoeic	Face	Slow	Scar-like plaque	Yellowish	Undefined telangiectasia
Metaphysical or basosquamous	Face	Rapid	Plaque + metastases	Yellowish	Undefined

their clinical aspect does not differ much from other BCCs. However it grows fast, has a destructive capacity and produces metastases.

Metatypical BCCs share uncharacteristic pathological features. These lesions frequently show a morphoeic aspect, and an intermediate histological pattern between squamous cell and BCC.

The histologic morphology of BCC can be divided into four patterns: nodular, superficial, metatypical (basosquamous), and morphea form (sclerosing).

1. Nodular BCC clinically presents as a raised, well-defined, smooth, pearly papule with associated telangiectasias. Nodular BCC is the most common type, accounting for upto 75% of all BCC.
2. Superficial BCC (10% of cases) present as discrete, well-defined, slightly raised plaques.
3. Morpheaform BCC accounts for 2% of all BCC. Examination shows an indurated plaque with a waxy-to-yellow appearance, ill-defined borders, sclerosis, and histologically irregular growth patterns.
4. The metatypical BCC is a histologic subtype with features of squamous differentiation.

Treatment of BCC depends on the size, location, and histologic pattern of the tumor. For most small nodular BCC in sites where tissue conservation is not an issue, electrodesiccation and curettage produce cure rates of approximately 90%. For large tumors, tumors near a free margin (lip, nasal ala, eyelid), or tumors located over embryologic fusion planes, excisional or Mohs micrographic surgery is the treatment of choice. BCC is radiosensitive, and radiation therapy is a treatment option.

SQUAMOUS CELL CARCINOMA

SCC is the second most common cutaneous malignancy. Lifetime probability of developing an SCC of 1.5% to 11%. Strong correlation between UV radiation and SCC development. The incidence of SCC increases with age, lighter skin type, and living at latitudes closer to the equator. A strong association with P_{53} gene defects is reported.

Eighty percent of SCC occur on the face, head and neck with some variation between the sexes. The nose and lower legs are most commonly affected in women and the nose and ears in men.

Diseases associated with an increased risk of SCC are burns, erythema ab igne, osteomyelitis, chronic ulcers, discoid lupus erythematosus, immune suppression, xeroderma pigmentosum, albinism, epidermolysis bullosa dystrophica, dyskeratosis congenita, and epidermodysplasia verruciformis. Radiation, cyclosporine, psoralen and ultraviolet. A phototherapy, polycyclic hydrocarbon, human papillomavirus, and arsenic exposure are some of the causative factors.

Surgical excision is the treatment of choice. Radiation therapy is a treatment option for patients who decline surgery, who have extensive involvement at the time of surgery, or who are not surgical candidates.

KERATOACANTHOMA

KA is a common, distinctive cutaneous tumor that is believed to arise from the hair follicle. KA occurs mainly on sun-exposed skin, with the majority located on the face, forearms and hands.

Men predominate with a ratio of 1:1 to 3:1. The occurrence on sun-exposed skin and presence in patients with xeroderma pigmentosum suggest UV radiation as a causative agent.

KA have **three distinct clinical stages**: proliferation, maturation, and involution. This three-stage cycle is believed to reflect the anagen, catagen, and telogen phases of hair growth, from which KA are suspected to arise.

It begins as a firm, hemispheric, smooth papule. The cutaneous border is skin tone to slightly erythematous with fine telangiectasias. During maturation, the KA becomes dome-shaped and develops a central umbilicated keratinous core.

The **histologic architectural features are diagnostic**. A keratin-filled core, epidermal lip, and glassy-appearing keratinocytes are classic.

The metastatic potential of KA should be negligible. Treatment of histologically confirmed KA prevents further enlargement and invasion into vital structures and is associated with a high cure rate.

PAGET'S DISEASE

PD is a nonsquamous intraepithelial neoplasia. Mammary and extramammary forms exist. PD is rare and may be a cutaneous marker for underlying malignancy. It is believed that Paget's cells are, in essence, ductal carcinoma cells that have migrated along the basement membrane to the epidermis.

Mammary PD is the presenting sign of breast cancer in 0.5% to 4.3% of patients. Mammary PD is extremely rare in the first three decades of life with a peak incidence between 50 and 60 years.

Extramammary PD is most commonly found on the vulva, followed by the anogenital and axillary regions. Pruritus, burning, pain, and tenderness are early and prominent symptoms with extramammary PD.

The **histology of mammary and extramammary PD is similar.** Paget's cells are large rounded or ovoid cells located in the epidermis. They have pale cytoplasm, large nucleoli, and enlarged pleomorphic hyperchromatic nuclei. They are found as single cells, nests, or acini or may replace the full thickness of the epidermis.

Because PD is a cutaneous intraepithelial neoplasm indicating an underlying cancer, treatment is directed at the primary neoplasm.

MERKEL CELL CARCINOMA

Merkel cells are thought to function as a receptor of mechanical stimuli and as a target for mechanosensory nerves during fetal development. The Merkel cell is found on mucous membranes and glabrous and hair-bearing skin with highest frequency in acral areas.

Merkel cells are located in or near the basal layer of the epidermis. They are difficult to differentiate from melanocytes, Langerhans' cells, and lymphocytes using light microscopy. Electron microscopy of MCC demonstrates distinct cytoplasmic membrane-bound spherical electron-dense core granules.

MCC has a predilection for sun-exposed sites on white skin. Fifty percent occur on the head and neck (with 20% in the periocular region) and 40% on the trunk.

MCC usually consists of painless, indurated, solitary dermal nodules measuring 2 to 4 mm.

MCC is an aggressive tumor with metastases to regional lymph nodes noted on initial diagnosis in 12% to 15% of cases. Surgical excision is the treatment of choice for primary tumors. MCCs are radiosensitive, and radiation therapy should be considered for all patients.

DERMATOFIBROSARCOMA PROTUBERANS

DFSP is a locally aggressive fibroblastic tumor of the dermis. DFSP is found on the trunk (50% to 60%), proximal extremities (20% to 30%), and the head and neck (10% to 15%).

DFSP is a slow, relentlessly enlarging malignancy.

Clinically, DFSP presents as an asymptomatic indurated red-brown or violaceous plaque. A solitary lesion is the rule. DFSP has the histology of a well-differentiated fibrosarcoma.

Treatment for DFSP is adequate surgical excision. The literature suggests that Mohs micrographic surgery is the treatment of choice for DFSP.

SEBACEOUS CARCINOMA

The ocular adnexa contain five types of sebaceous glands, including the meibomian and Zeis glands. **Ectopic sebaceous glands (Fordyce's condition)** are found on the vermilion border of the lip and the buccal mucosa.

Seventy-five percent of all SC are located on the eyelid. Ocular SC represents 1% to 5.5% of all eyelid malignancies. **The incidence of ocular SC ranks fourth, behind BCC, SCC, and malignant melanoma. SC of the upper lid is two to three times more common than lower lid lesion (greater number of meibomian glands in the upper lid),** seen in patients 60 to 80 years of age. Incidence of ocular SC appears to be higher in women (57% to 77%) and in Asians. Sites of extraocular SC include the head and neck, external genitalia, parotid and submandibular glands, external auditory canal, trunk and upper extremity.

SC is an aggressive malignancy.

Surgical intervention is the preferred treatment.

SEBORRHEIC KERATOSES

Seborrheic keratoses are common, **benign neoplasms** of keratinocytes. With age, nearly everyone develops some of them.

Clinical Features

Early lesions appear as hyperpigmented macules. They often appear first on the torso and tend to be ovoid or elongated with orientation along skin cleavage lines. They generally begin to appear after the third decade of life. Fully developed lesions take the form of waxy, stuck-on plaques, which are hyperkeratotic and often hyperpigmented.

Variants

A variant termed stucco keratoses is multiple skin-colored or hypopigmented, slightly elevated, uniform small plaques that tend to occur symmetrically on the lower legs. The sign of Leser-Trelat is the sudden appearance of multiple seborrheic keratoses; it is a sign of internal malignancy.

Relevant Clinical Encounters

Inflamed Seborrheic Keratosis: The presentation is often that of changing mole. Sometimes owing to chronic low-level trauma and sometimes spontaneously, seborrheic keratoses may become inflamed; redness, crusting, erosion, itching,

Seborrheic Keratosis Versus Melanocytic Lesion

It may be difficult or impossible to distinguish a flat seborrheic keratosis from a lentigo maligna (melanoma in situ on sun-damaged skin). Both are large, hyperpigmented macules.

Treatment

Treatment directed at removing the involved epithelium without disturbing the underlying dermis; in this way, scarring may be avoided or minimized. Cryotherapy is effective for all but the thickest, most hyperkeratotic lesions, but in more darkly pigmented skin, hypopigmentation may result from this treatment.

DERMATOFIBROMAS

Dermatofibromas are common neoplasms that are most typically firm, deep-seated, nodules often with some hyperpigmentation.

Clinical Features

Dermatofibromas are most commonly seen on the legs. They are firm, deep-seated dermal nodules, often with some hyperpigmentation. It is thought that they result from minor localized trauma generally asymptomatic. A useful diagnostic sign of dermatofibromas is their tendency to dimple or indent on lateral pressure.

Relevant Clinical Encounter

KELOIDS

Keloids are nodular growths of fibrous tissue, often following tissue trauma.

Clinical Features

The tendency to form keloids may be familial.

Keloids tend to be nodules or plaques. Earlobe keloids may be protuberant or pedunculated. The plaque-type lesions may spread out in an irregular shape. The epidermis overlying keloids is smooth and shiny.

Relevant Clinical Encounter

Diagnosis is rarely a problem with these lesions. Dermatologists commonly treat keloids with intralesional corticosteroid injections repeated at intervals. If surgical excision of a keloid is planned, the lesion should be pretreated with intralesional corticosteroids for a number of months before the surgery.

CHERRY (ADULT ACQUIRED) HEMANGIOMAS

Cherry hemangiomas are common vascular growths that tend to accumulate on the trunk and extremities.

Clinical Features

The lesions are generally 1 to 3 mm, nonblanching, dark red, rounded, smooth-surfaced, asymptomatic papules in random distribution.

Relevant Clinical Encounter

A traumatized hemangioma may bleed or may thrombose and thus darken to a deep purple or even black color.

Treatment

Most lesions do not need treatment.

CHILDHOOD HEMANGIOMAS

Two common variants of early-onset hemangiomas are the strawberry hemangioma and the naevus flammeus.

Clinical Features

Strawberry hemangiomas may be present at birth or may appear during the first few months of life. They tend to begin as flat patches and rapidly grow for several months to a year. They may remain stable for some time but nearly always involute during preschool years. Bleeding on minor trauma is expected.

Naevus flammeus or port-wine stains are macular red or pink macules most commonly seen on the back of the neck. They are common in childhood. They rarely produce symptoms and often are unappreciated by patients. Lesions in the trigeminal nerve distribution suggest the Sturge-Weber syndrome, in which there is involvement of the underlying leptomeninges with a number of neurologic consequences. High incidence of spontaneous resolution of strawberry hemangiomas in the first few years of life, and the final appearance of the involved area is likely to be better from such natural healing than from any medical intervention.

Almost complete healing by (9 months).

Treatment

Rarely, there may be uncontrollable bleeding. More rarely, there may be platelet sequestration with hematologic consequences **(Kasabach-Merritt syndrome).** More commonly, treatment is considered if the lesions are interfering with a vital anatomic structure, such as the nose or eye. Specific treatments include surgical (excision, cautery, cryosurgery or laser ablation) or medical (oral or intralesional steroids) options.

For naevus flammeus, the question of treatment centers on the degree of disfigurement produced, typically by facial lesions.

ACROCHORDONS

Commonly termed skin tags, acrochordons are fleshy papillomatous growths that tend to occur in intertriginous sites.

Clinical Features

Lesions may be skin colored or hyperpigmented. They tend to cluster at the sides of the neck, in the axillary region, and in the inguinal crease. Obesity is a predisposing factor.

Acrochordons are generally pedunculated; they are composed of an outpouching of normal dermis with an epidermis that is normal or hyperplastic.

Treatment

Generally, they are electrodesiccated or simply snipped off.

CYSTS

The most common type of cutaneous cyst is the epidermoid or epidermal inclusion cyst.

Clinical Features

Epidermoid cysts are firm, round and generally mobile. If they are superficially placed in the skin, they are whitish.

Relevant Clinical Encounter

Often cysts of this type come to medical attention when they become inflamed. Such lesions are red, tender and edematous. The contents of an epidermoid cyst are cheesy keratin.

Treatment

Ruptured cysts may be treated by local heat, drainage and antibiotics. If the cyst is firm and not amenable to draining, intralesional corticosteroid injections help reduce inflammation quickly.

Variants

Milia are small, superficially located epidermoid cysts. They are most common on the face. They may occur in the context of acne vulgaris, sun damage, or after trauma or certain skin diseases.

Pilar cysts are epithelial cysts that show histologic features of trichilemmal keratinization, a recapitulation of the pattern in the middle portion of the hair follicle. These lesions are most prevalent on the scalp. They are commonly multiple.

Glomus Tumour

- This arises within the glomus body, a neuromyoarterial receptor (the Sucquet-Hoyer canal)

that is sensitive to temperature variations and regulates arterial blood flow.
- These tumors, more common on the fingers and toes and beneath the nail plate.
- Usually seen in young adults between the third and fourth decade of life.
- They can be solitary of multiple.
- Classically presents as solitary, small, blue–red nodules on the hand (nail bed) that are characteristically associated with paroxysmal pain often elicited by changes in temperature.
- Simple excision—treatment of choice.

Premalignant Epidermal Tumours

Actinic keratosis (senile or solar keratosis):
- Most common premalignant skin tumour.
- These lesions occur in sun-damaged skin of elderly people having light complexion.
- Clinically, these lesions are rounds to irregular keratotic papules surrounded by erythema.
- The principal sites are the back of the hands, forearm and face.
- Squamous cell carcinoma can develop from actinic keratosis.
- Histologically there may be vacuolization of keratinocytes with numerous mitotic figures seen involving the lower layers of the epidermis (carcinoma in situ).
- Treatment medical—topical tretinoin and topical 5 fluorouracil and surgical—curettage, electrodesiccation and cryotherapy.

Erythroplasia of Queyrat

- This condition affect uncircumcised males.
- Seen in the fifth and sixth decades of life.
- The lesions present as sharply defined brightly erythematous and velvetty plaque with moist glistening or granular surface over the glans penis.
- Differentiated from benign inflammatory dermatoses such as psoriasis, lichen planus, Zoon's plasma cell balanitis and fixed drug eruptions.
- Treatment with topical 5- fluorouracil produces satisfactory results.

Bowen's Disease

- Refers to cutaneous plaques of intraepidermal squamous cell carcinoma.
- Chronic sunlight exposure, inorganic arsenicals are important etiologic factors.
- Clinically lesions of Bowen's disease appear as solitary, sharply defined, round or oval to irregular erythematous psoriasiform or eczematous plaque.
- Ulceration is a sign of development of invasive carcinoma.
- Histology shows proliferating atypical squamous cells through the full thickness of the epidermis ("wind-blown appearance").
- The most effective treatment for Bowen's disease is surgical excision.

Cutaneous Horn (Cornu Cutaneum)

- Cutaneous horn (cornu cutaneum) is the term coined for horny skin excrescence, which in its form and consistency resembles an animal horn in miniature.
- The paramount consideration while making a clinical diagnosis is the height of the keratotic mass (at least one half of its largest diameter). It is reaction pattern of exaggerated hyperkeratosis and is rarely, if ever seen now-a-days. Its association with various dermatoses may be informative.
- The important issue is not the horn itself which is dead keratin, but rather the nature of underlying condition, which may be benign (seborrheic keratosis, viral warts, histiocytoma, inverted follicular keratosis, verrucous epidermal naevus, organoid naevus, ichthyosis hystrix, palmoplantar trichilemmal cysts, lichen planus, corn and calluses, scar, molluscum contagiosum), premalignant (solar keratosis, arsenical keratoses, Bowen's disease) or

malignant (squamous cell carcinoma, rarely, basal cell carcinoma, metastatic renal carcinoma, granular cell tumor, sebaceous carcinoma of Kaposi's sarcoma).

- In the majority of cases, these horns are benign.
- Most commonly, they are single and arise from a seborrheic keratoses lesion.
- They are encountered most frequently on the face and scalp, but may occur on the hands, penis and eyelids.

Kaposi's Sarcoma

- Kaposi's sarcomas (KS) are multisystem vascular neoplasms, characterized by mucocutaneous violaceous lesions and oedema as well as involvement of nearly any organ.
- Human herpes virus type 8 has been implicated in the pathogenesis.
- KS have been classified into four types—classical type, African-endemic type, iatrogenic immunosuppression associated type and HIV associated type (Epidemic type).
- Presents as ecchymotic macules, which become purple and brownish with hemosiderotic halo. The lesion evolves into patches, plaques and nodules and are often arranged parallel to skin tension lines.
- Classical KS lesion occurs on the leg in the mean age of 60 years age.
- Oral lesion can be the first manifestation of KS in the majority of cases, especially in those having underlying HIV infection.
- Histologically, a characteristic sign of KS is the presence of solid cords and fascicles of oval or spindle shaped cells arranged between the jagged vascular channels. These structures dissect the collagen bundles of the entire dermis, leaving a spongy network of collagen. This biphasic tumor morphology, exhibiting both angiomatous and solid tumor patterns, changes to a clear-cut sarcomatous morphology.
- Modalities of management include—radiation and chemotherapy.

Mycosis Fungoides

Mycosis fungoides is a form of cutaneous T-cell lymphoma (CTCL):

- It is a chronic, slowly progressive disease that evolves from patches (Patch stage) to plaques (plaque stage) and subsequently nodules (tumour stage).
- Pruritus is a prominent symptom.
- The lesions coalesce and may ulcerate, leading to deep ulcers.
- Prognosis depends upon the TNM staging.
- **Diagnosis:** Clinically lesions can be confused with eczema and psoriasis. Histopathology reveals atypical lymphocytes infiltrating the epidermis without spongiosis (epidermotropism). The pathognomonic feature is presence of pautraler microabscess (collection of atypical lymphocytes in the epidermis). The dermis has dense monomorphous lyphomononuclear infiltrate with grenz zone.
- **Treatment:** It depends on the stage of the disease. Chemotherapy, retinoids, electron beam therapy, photochemotherapy etc have been used.

Sezary Syndrome

Sezary syndrome is a rare special variant of cutaneous T-cell lymphoma characterized by a triad of features—erythroderma, peripheral lymphadenopathy and infiltrates of atypical cells in the skin and blood.

- It occurs in people older than 60 years and more commonly in males.
- There is generalized erythroderma with diffuse hyperkeratosis of palms and soles and diffuse hair loss.
- Peripheral smear shows more than 10% atypical lymphocytic cells in the blood.
- Treatment is chemotherapy combined with electron beam therapy or photochemotherapy.

MULTIPLE CHOICE QUESTIONS

1. Sutton's naevus is usually a benign melanocytic naevus but may be a:
A. Neuroid naevus
B. Blue naevus
C. Neuro fibroma
D. Primary or secondary malignant melanoma
E. All of the above

2. The single most important factor that determines prognosis, treatment, and follow-up recommendations in melanoma is:
A. Breslow depth of invasion
B. Clark level
C. Histologic subtype
D. Radial growth phase

3. Koebner's phenomenon is not seen in:
A. Psoriasis vulgaris
B. Lichen planus
C. Basal cell carcinoma
D. Verruca plana

4. The development of numerous pruritic seborrhoeic keratosis as a manifestation of a systemic malignancy is:
A. Monsters's sign
B. Lesèr trelat sign
C. Lichtheim sign
D. Mirchamp sign

5. Electron beam is often the choice treatment in:
A. Neurodermatitis
B. Lymphosarcoma
C. Mycosis fungoides
D. Multiple myeloma

6. Pyoderma gangrenosum, especially if superficial and bulbous should cause one to look for:
A. Leukaemia
B. Lupus erythematosus
C. Chronic real disease
D. Diabetes mellitus

7. Which of the following indicates malignant change in naevus?
A. Itching
B. Change in color
C. Increase in size
D. Appearance of pain

8. True about rodent ulcer *except*:
A. Blood spread common
B. Local invasion
C. Healing and then recurrence
D. Response to radiotherapy

9. Malignant melanoma usually arises from:
A. Hairy mole
B. Epidermal naevus
C. Junctional naevus
D. Dermal naevus

10. Keratin pearls are seen histopathologically in:
A. Squamous cell carcinoma of skin
B. Basal cell carcinoma of skin
C. Keratoacanthoma
D. Melanoma

1 E 2 A 3 C 4 B 5 C 6 A 7 C 8 A 9 C 10 A

11. **Which of the following is probably the treatment of choice for dermatofibrosarcoma protuberans?**
    A. Total skin electron beam therapy
    B. Liquid nitrogen cryosurgery
    C. Electrodesiccation and curettage
    D. Mohs micrographic surgery

12. **In Bazex syndrome there is associated malignancy of:**
    A. Thyroid
    B. Laryngopharynx
    C. Pituitary
    D. Colon

13. **Which of the following is the treatment of choice for lentigo maligna (in situ melanoma)?**
    A. Radiation therapy
    B. Cryosurgery combined with laser therapy
    C. Electrodesiccation and curettage
    D. Surgical resection with margin control

14. **The loss of which of the following T-cell antigens supports the diagnosis of mycosis fungoides?**
    A. CD 4   B. CD 7
    C. CD 25   D. CD 3

15. **Which of the following conditions has been reported to progress to mycosis fungoides?**
    A. Guttate parapsoriasis
    B. Large-plaque parapsoriasis
    C. Actinic reticuloid
    D. Chronic photocontact dermatitis

16. **The most common type of carcinoma cutis in women originates from the:**
    A. Esophagus
    B. Larynx
    C. Lung
    D. Breast

17. **The most common location for trichoepithelioma is the:**
    A. Neck
    B. Scalp
    C. Face
    D. Back

18. **Mycosis cells are altered ....:**
    A. T lymphocytes
    B. Monocytes
    C. B lymphocytes
    D. Eosinophils

19. **The following is a premycotic lesion:**
    A. Acne vermoulanate
    B. Alopecia mucinosa
    C. Bowenoid papulosis
    D. Lymphocytoma cutis

20. **Which of the following does not have lymphatic spread?**
    A. Squamous cell carcinoma
    B. Basal cell carcinoma
    C. Malignant melanoma
    D. Adenocarcinoma

21. **Margins of squamous cell carcinoma are:**
    A. Inverted
    B. Everted
    C. Rolled
    D. Undermined

22. **True about rodent ulcer *except*:**
    A. Blood spread common
    B. Local invasion
    C. Healing and then recurrence
    D. Response to radiotherapy

11 D **12** B **13** D **14** B **15** B **16** D **17** C **18** A **19** B **20** B **21** B **22** A

Chapter 18

Systemic Disease and Skin

1. Skin in Liver Disease

As a general rule, the cutaneous findings are non-specific and may be absent even in the presence of severe liver dysfunction.

- **Pruritus** is the most common symptom and may be mild or severe. In obstructive jaundice, it is due to presence of bile salts in skin. Therapeutic response to antihistamines is limited and oral cholestyramine, 8-12 g daily may give relief. There may be urticaria and serum sickness like picture. There may be a yellowish hue of sclera and soft palate due to icterus.
- **Telangiectasias** producing paper money skin, palmar erythema, purpuric lesions, varicose veins may be evident. Diffuse muddy grey hypermelanosis, more in the sun-exposed areas may develop Biliary cirrhosis may be associated with **Xanthomas.**
- Nails may show clubbing, white flat nails and white bands. Body hair becomes sparse and males may develop female pubic hair pattern.
- **Gianotti Crosti syndrome** may be associated with Hepatitis C and B infection respectively. In addition erythema multiforme erythema nodosum may be presenting features.

2. Skin in Renal Disease

- These are also only of limited diagnostic value. Uraemic patients have a dry, scaly skin.
- There may be severe pruritus in one third cases.

In intractable itching UVB radiation, UVA, oral cholestyramine and activated charcoal may be beneficial.

- Purpura and delayed wound healing may be seen.
- Anaemia is evident and muddy brown hyper-pigmentation can develop.
- Metastatic calcification, perforating dermatoses acquired porphyrias may manifest. Some patients develop uraemic neuropathy. Upto 40% patients with renal failure can develop gynae comastia which may be reversed on a low phosphorus diet.

3. Skin in Endocrine Disorders

- Hyperthyroidism Cutaneous symptoms of hyperthyroidism are thickening of epidermis and soft, velvetty, dry skin.
- Increased skin temperature due to high sympathetic activity.
- Palmar erythema and flushing of face.
- Increased sweating (especially palms and soles).
- Fast nail growth with distal onycholysis.
- Diffuse Addisonian hyperpigmentation.
- Diffuse thinning of scalp hair.
- Acropachy.
- Pretibial myxoedema—Skin coloured, oedematous pretibial plaques or nodules with prominent hair follicles may develop on the shins or abdomen. The lesions may be nodular, diffuse

or elephantiasic. Treatment with topical steroids or surgery may be successful.

a. Hypothyroidism

The skin changes are:

- Pale, cold, scaly, wrinkled skin.
- Puffy oedema of hands, face, eyelids and carotenaemia.
- Reduced sweating with eczema craquele xanthomatosis.
- Purpura, ecchymoses, punctate telangiectasias on fingertips, delayed wound healing.
- Brittle and striated nails.
- Presence of coarse sparse scalp hair, loss of lateral eyebrows and axillary pubic hair.

b. Hypercorticism

- **Skin in Cushing's syndrome:** There is excess production or supply of glucocorticoid hormone.
- The patients develop moon faces, buffalo lump.
- Purlish striae, telangiectasias, osteoporosis can be seen.

c. Skin in Hirsutism

- Acne may be pronounced.
- In females male pattern baldness may manifest.
- 10% patients of noniatrogenic disease have Addisonian like pigmentation.

d. Skin in Diabetes Mellitus

- Infections.
- Poorly controlled diabetes may be associated with increased staphylococcal pyodermas especially furunculosis, vulvovaginal candidiasis, erythrasma and epidermophytosis.
- Particularly, infection of foot is dangerous, due to associated neuropathy and vascular compromise trophic ulcer can occur.
- Xanthomatosis is seen due to hyperlipidaemia, mainly involving triglyceride and cholesterol.
- Due to chronic degenerative complications there may be diabetic dermopathy, which presents as brownish atrophic circumscribed.
- Lesions on lower extremities.
- Reddening of face (rubeosis faciel) and erysipelas like areas on lower legs and feet with or without necrosis.
- Spontaneous bullae formation on feet which heal in several weeks.
- Thickened waxy skin over dorsa of hand, stiff joints and scleredema.
- Adultorum; which is induration of skin beginning from neck that does not pit on pressure.
- Autonomic disturbances may accompany sensory neuropathy.

4. Disorders Common in Diabetes

Necrobiosis Lipoidica Diabeticorum— This occurs in 0.3 percent diabetics. It begins as a dusky red nodule, which becomes an irregular plaque, brownish yellow with red margins and associated atrophy with telangiectasias. It is asymptomatic but painful ulcers may develop. 10% patients have normal glucose tolerance tests. Treatment modalities include topical and intralesional steroids, clofazimine, nicotinamide, aspirin and pentoxifyllin. Acanthosis Nigricans—Velvetty, papillomatous hyperpigmented plaques develop in axillae, groins, neck, flexor creases. It may occur due to insulin resistance. Granuloma annulare, vitiligo, Kyrle's disease, reactive perforating collagenosis, skin tags have all been seen to occur more frequently in diabetes.

MULTIPLE CHOICE QUESTIONS

1. Lupus perino is seen in:
A. Porphyria
B. Sarcoidosis
C. Tuberous sclerosis
D. Pellagra

2. Acanthosis nigricans is indicative of:
A. Internal malignancy
B. Endocrine disorder
C. Bloom's syndrome
D. Pigmentation of face, neck etc.
E. All of the above

3. Pathergy test is positive in:
A. Psoriasis vulgaris
B. Pemphigus vulgaris
C. Bechet's syndrome
D. Reiter's syndrome

4. 'Cassals necklace' is a feature of:
A. Acrodermatitis enteropathica
B. Niacin deficiency
C. Ceruloplasmin deficiency
D. Essential fatty acid toxicity

5. Beaded margins of eyelids is a characteristic feature of:
A. Granuloma annulare
B. Leprosy
C. Erythema annulare centrifugum
D. Lipoid proteiniosis

6. Langer's lines are seen in:
A. Lichen planus
B. Atopic dermatitis
C. Psoriasis
D. Normal persons

7. Internal malignancy is/are frequently associated with:
A. Erythema gyratum repens
B. Erythema chronicum migrans
C. Erythema annulare centrifugum
D. All of the above

8. Difference in skin color between caucasoids and Negro in spite of having equal number of melanocytes is due to:
A. Greater production of melanosomes per melanocyte in Negroes
B. Melanosomes are larger in Negroes
C. High degree of dispersion of melanin in keratinocytes in Negroes
D. All of the above
E. None of the above

9. All of the following hyperpigmentation disorders are due to increased dermal melanocytes *except*:
A. Mongolian spot
B. Naevus of ota
C. Naevus of ITO
D. Lentigines

10. Naevus depigmentosus all true *except*:
A. Usually presents in second year of life
B. Lesions may be multiple
C. Lesions may be in dermatomal or whorled pattern
D. Defect in transfer of melanosomes to keratinocytes has been postulated

1 B 2 E 3 C 4 B 5 D 6 D 7 A 8 C 9 D 10 B

11. All true of berloque dermatitis *except*:

A. Caused by beugamot oil contained in perfumes

B. Wavelengths between 290-320 nn are involved

C. Deep brown pigmentation along the trickling of perfume

D. The pigmentation fades after weeks or months

12. Treatment of choice for facial port- wine stain:

A. Argon laser

B. Tunable pulsed dye laser

C. Nd-YAG laser

D. Ruby laser

13. The following diseases are aggravated by exposure to sunlight *except*:

A. Freckles

B. Melanocytic naevus

C. Xeroderma pigmentosum

D. Discoid lupus erythematosus

14. Pruritus of renal disease:

A. Psychogenic

B. Indicates probable renal malignancy

C. Related to level of azotemia

D. Occurs in chronic pyelonephritis and chronic glomerulonephritis but not in acute nephritis

15. The following are correct statements concerning steroids used topically:

A. Halogenation decreases topical activity

B. Thinning of epidermis may occur

C. Thinning of dermis may occur

D. Systemic side-effects commonly occur

E. The rate of epidermal turnover is increased

16. Progressive pigmented purpuric dermatosis is also called:

A. Sweet syndrome

B. Darier's disease

C. Hailey-Hailey disease

D. Schamberg's disease

17. Necrobiosis lipoidica diabeticorum is most marked on:

A. Forearms

B. Face

C. Front of legs

D. Back of legs

18. Poor prognostic indicators for vitiligo are all *except*:

A. Long duration

B. Young age of onset

C. Leukotrichia

D. Acrofacial vitiligo

19. Half and half nails are seen in:

A. Liver disease

B. Chronic renal failure

C. COPD

D. SLE

20. All of the following disease frequency involve both the kidney and skin *except*:

A. Polyarteritis nodosa

B. Wegner's granulomatosis

C. Erythema nodosum

D. Henoch-Schönlein purpura

21. Dermatoses associated with internal malignancy include all *except*:

A. Acanthosis nigricans

B. Erythema gyratum repens

C. Erythroderma

D. Ichthyosis

E. Vitiligo

22. First line treatment of keloid is:

A. Wide excision

B. Intralesional corticosteroids

C. Radiotherapy

D. Local steroids

---

11 D 12 B 13 B 14 C 15 B,C 16 D 17 C 18 B 19 A,B 20 C 21 E 22 B

23. Poliosis is:
- A. Localised patch of white hair
- B. Skin changes in poliomyelitis
- C. Premature greying of hair
- D. Localised patch of baldness

24. Which laser is colored blue green?
- A. Argon
- B. CO_2
- C. Ruby
- D. YAG

25. Which laser is selectively absorbed?
- A. Argon
- B. CO_2
- C. Ruby
- D. YAG

26. True about Kveim's test is:
- A. Subcutaneous test
- B. Highly specific for sarcoidosis
- C. Dextrose extract from sarcoid tissue used
- D. Has some degree of prognostic value

27. Berloque dermatitis is due to contact with:
- A. Metals
- B. Dyes
- C. Food
- D. Photosensitizing agents

28. The syndrome of intestinal polyposis pigmentation of skin around the mouth and oral mucosa is found in:
- A. Toni Fanconi syndrome
- B. Peutz-Jeghar's syndrome
- C. Reiter's syndrome
- D. Carcinoid syndrome

29. De Morgan's spots most often require:
- A. Local keratolytic agents
- B. Local steroids
- C. Local retinoids
- D. No treatment

30. All are proposed etiological hypothesis for vitiligo *except*:
- A. Autoimmune
- B. Self-destruct
- C. Neurogenic
- D. Composite
- E. Psychogenic

31. Following conditions have increased association with vitiligo *except:*
- A. Thyroiditis
- B. Pernicious anaemia
- C. Hepatitis
- D. Morphea
- E. Diabetes

32. The following is true of Meirowsky phenomenon *except*:
- A. Best observed in hyperpigmented skin
- B. Most effective induced by UVA
- C. It is a delayed tanning reaction
- D. It is transient

33. PUVA lentigines most commonly seen with:
- A. Skin type I, II
- B. Skin type III, IV
- C. Skin type V, VI
- D. Skin type II, III
- E. Skin type IV, V

34. All true about albinism *except*:
- A. Most forms are autosomal recessive
- B. Defect in enzyme tyrosinase
- C. Melanocytes are completely absent in the skin
- D. Melanocytes are normal in number but the melanocytes synthesize inadequate amounts of melanin
- E. Depigmented or hypopigmented skin and hair, nystagmus, photophobia and decreased visual activity

23 A 24 A 25 C 26 D 27 D 28 B 29 D 30 E 31 C 32 C 33 A
34 C

35. **Piebaldism—all true *except*:**
  A. Depigmented patches of skin present at birth
  B. White forelock
  C. Islands of normal or hypermelanotic skin occur in the white areas
  D. Autosomal recessive inheritance

36. **The primary event causing Kyrle's disease is:**
  A. Perforation of the epidermis
  B. Abnormally fast keratinization
  C. Increased rate of cell proliferation
  D. All of the above

37. **Malignant acanthosis nigricans is most commonly caused by:**
  A. Lymphoma
  B. Squamous cell carcinoma
  C. Adenocarcinoma
  D. Mycosis fungoides

38. **Pseudocanthosis nigricans is seen in:**
  A. Endocrine disorders
  B. Metabolic disorders
  C. Abdominal cancers
  D. Obese

39. **Chemicals like monebenzyle ether of hydroquinone cause skin depigmentation by:**
  A. Inhibiting tyrosinase
  B. Destroying melanocytes
  C. Preventing transfer of melonosomes
  D. Decreasing melanin synthesis

40. **Cafe-au-lait macules (CALM) are associated with all *except*:**
  A. Neurofibromatosis
  B. McCune-Albright syndrome
  C. Fanconi's syndrome
  D. Acropigmentation of kitamura

41. **All modalities are used to treat vitiligo *except*:**
  A. PUVA therapy
  B. Potent topical steroids
  C. Punch grafting
  D. Tattooing
  E. Laser
  F. Disorders of keratinization

42. **The wavelength of light responsible for most cases of polymorphic light sensitive eruption is:**
  A. 290-350 nm
  B. 320-380 nm
  C. 400-700 nm
  D. 700-800 nm

43. **Erythema ab igne is caused by:**
  A. Repeated friction
  B. Repeated and prolonged exposure to heat
  C. Repeated and prolonged exposure to cold
  D. Prolonged exposure to sunlight

44. **The concentration of hydroquinone for treating chloasma should be:**
  A. Less than 1%
  B. 1-2%
  C. 2-5 %
  D. 10%

45. **Lichen spinulosus is least common on:**
  A. Abdomen
  B. Buttocks
  C. Legs
  D. Arms

46. **Blue naevus is most common on:**
  A. Arms
  B. Chest
  C. Face
  D. Legs

35 D 36 A 37 C 38 D 39 B 40 D 41 E 42 A 43 B 44 C 45 D 46 C

47. Lupus pernio is seen in:
A. Porphyria
B. Sarcoidosis
C. Tuberous sclerosis
D. Pellagra

48. The following skin diseases are associated with internal malignancy:
A. Erythema nodosum
B. Dermatomyositis
C. Pyoderma gangrenosum
D. Acanthosis nigricans
E. Acquired ichthyosis

49. Most common cutaneous manifestation of viral hepatitis other than icterus and pruritus follows:
A. Urticaria
B. Purpura
C. Morbiliform erythema
D. Scarlatiniform erythema

47 B 48 A-E 49 A

Chapter 19

Ages of Men and Their Dermatoses

Dermatoses of Puberty and Adolescence

These include:

- *Acne vulgaris*—This is a common dermatosis seen during puberty due to associated hormonal changes which lead to an increase sebum production. The psychological aspect of this disease is profound.
- *Acne excorie and neurotic excoriation*—Commonly seen in adolescent girls who are concious about body image. Leads to scarring.
- *Self mutilation and dermatitis artefacta*—An artefactural skin disease caused entirely by the actions of the fully aware patients on the skin, hair, nails or mucosae. There is no rational motive for this behaviour.
- *Seborrheic dermatitis*—Commonly seen due to an increase in sebum production. Malassezia furfur has been implicated.
- *Pityriasis versicolor*—Commonly seen in the summer months. Response to anti-fungals is good.

Hyperhidrosis, axillary bromhidrosis, Fox-Fordyce disease and polymorphic light eruption are the other commonly seen conditions during this period.

Dermatoses of Pregnancy

Pregnancy is characterized by the advent of a new endocrine organ (the placenta). Placenta produces steroid hormones like estrogens, progesterone and proteins hormones including HCG, HPL and HCT. Hence, there is a profound physiological endocrine upheaval leading to cutaneous changes which can be divided into physiological and pathological.

Physiological Changes

1. *Pigmentary changes:* There is a generalized increase in skin pigmentation more so over the nipples, areolae, genital areas and the midline of the abdominal wall. Chloasmal pigmentation is seen in about 70% of women which may fade completely after parturition or persist. Also, an increase in the size, activity and also, number of melanocyte naevi has been observed.
2. *Hair and nail changes:* Post partum alopecia and mild frontoparietal recession may occur. Brittle-ness of nail plate and distal onycholysis has been reported.
3. *Eccrine, apocrine and sebaceous gland activity:* There is increased frequency of miliaria although palmar sweating decreases. Fox-Fordyce disease usually improves in pregnancy, suggesting a reduced apocrine activity. Sebum excretion tends to increase during pregnancy and return to normal after delivery.

4. *Vascular changes:* Sustained high levels of circulating estrogens result in vascular spiders palmar erythema and haemangiomas all of which usually disappear post partum. Varicose veins and haemorrhoids are frequent complications of pregnancy. Gingival edema and pregnancy epulis are seen in around 80% of pregnant women as a result of the general increase in vascularity associated with high estrogen levels.
5. *Connective tissue:* Striae distensae and multiple skin tags are common features of most pregnancies.

Specific dermatoses of pregnancy include pemphigoid (herpes) gestationis, polymorphic erutpion of pregnancy, Prurigo of pregnancy (Besnier) and pruritic folliculitis of pregnancy. The less well-defined dermatosis include papular dermatitis of pregnancy, auto-immune progesterone dermatitis of pregnancy and prurigo annularis.

Pemphigoid Gestations

Incidence of 1 in 1,50,000 pregnancies has been reported. HLA mismatch between mother and fetus and auto-immunity due to association with other autoimmune disease like Grave's, vitiligos and alopecia areata has been implicated in the etiology. Clinical features include urticated papules, plaques, vesicles, target lesions and weals seen around the umbilicus in the second or third trimester, which later spread to involve the abdomen and thighs. Differential diagnosis includes pruritic urticarial papules and plaques of pregnancy, dermatitis herpetiformis and erythema multiforme. Treatment includes steroids (topical and systemic), anti histaminics, plasmapheresis and azathioprine.

Polymorphic Eruption of Pregnancy

Incidence of 1 in 240 pregnancies is reported. The eruption begins in third trimester, usually of first pregnancy. Aetiology is obscure. Clinically intensely itchy, urticated papules and plaques over the lines of striae which later spread to upper arms and thighs are seen. Treatment modalities include topical calamine or steroids and systemic sedative antihistamines.

Prurigo of Pregnancy

Incidence is 1 in 30 pregnancies. Usually begins between 25 and 30 weeks of gestation. Clinical features include multiple excoriated papules seen over the abdomen and on the extensor surfaces of the limbs. The lesions tend to persist throughout pregnancy and puerperium, but the pruritic element usually settles after birth. Treatment is symptomatic.

Pruritic Folliculitis of Pregnancy

Itchy, red, follicular papules strongly resembling steroid induced acne are seen beginning in the second or third trimester usually resolves within 2 weeks of delivery.

Increased incidence of infections like candidiasis, trichomoniasis, condylomata acuminata, pityrosporum folliculitis, herpes simplex and autoimmune disorders like lupus erythematosus and pemphigus are seen during pregnancy. Tumors like mycosis fungoides and neurofibromatosis also show increased frequency.

Dermatoses of Old Age

Pruritus

Itch may be localized or generalized and may or may not be accompanied by skin changes. An itchy elderly person should be carefully examined for primary cutaneous diseases like scabies, bullous pemphigoid, candidiasis, lichen sclerosus et atrophicus etc. Systemic causes like renal disease, cholestasis (especially chronic liver disease), thyroid disease, anaemia or cancer should also be ruled out. Treatment includes topical emollients and potent steroids, sedative systemic antihistaminics and to treat the underlying cause, if any.

Systemic diseases associated with pruritus

Renal disease
- Chronic renal failure

Hepatobiliary disease
- Intrahepatic cholestasis
- Primary biliary cirrhosis
- Pruritus gravidarum
- Sclerosing cholangitis
- Infectious hepatitis
- Drug induced cholestasis
- Extrahepatic biliary obstruction

Hematopoietic diseases
- Polycythemia vera
- Iron-deficiency anemia
- Hodgkin's disease
- Leukemias and Lymphomas
- Plasma cell dyscrasias
- Mycosis fungoides
- Mastocytosis

Metabolic and endocrine disorders
- Hyperthyroidism
- Hypothyroidism
- Diabetes mellitus
- Multiple endocrine neoplasia II (Sipple syndrome)
- Carcinoid syndrome

Neurologic disorders
- Multiple sclerosis
- Cerebral tumor
- Cerebral abscess
- Stroke

Malignancy

Miscellaneous conditions
- Acquired immunodeficiency syndrome (AIDS)
- Parasitosis
- Anorexia nervosa
- Advanced age
- Psychogenic disorders

Management of pruritus associated with chronic renal failure

Ultraviolet B (UVB) phototherapy twice weekly
Oral-activated charcoal 6 g daily
Cholestyramine 5 g twice daily
Naltrexone 50 mg daily
Ondansetron 4 mg twice daily
Topical capsaicin (if localized)
Encourage renal transplantation program enrolment

Management of pruritus associated with intrahepatic cholestasis

Cholestyramine 4 g once to three times daily
Rifampin 300-450 mg daily
Ultraviolet B (UVB) phototherapy twice weekly
Naltrexone 50 mg daily
Ondansetron 8 mg twice daily
Encourage liver transplantation program enrolment

Management of pruritus associated with polycythemia vera

Phlebotomy or chemotherapy to reduce red cell mass
Cyproheptadine 4 mg three times daily
Cimetidine 300 three times daily
Pizotifen 0.5 mg three times daily
Cholestyramine 4 mg three daily

Eczema Craquele

The dryness is often worse in winters. Changes are more pronounced on the legs. Treatment includes emollients and decreased use of soaps and detergents.

Seborrheic dermatitis, discoid eczema (Sulzberger Garbe disease) and gravitational eczema are commonly seen. Atopic dermatitis may occasionally be seen.

Contact dermatitis of irritant or allergic origin is considered to be less common. Marked secondary lichenification and chronic lichen simplex are often seen.

Bullous Disorders

Pemphigoid is much more frequent in the elderly than in other age groups.

Psoriasis

There is a distinct peak of onset of psoriasis in later life. Flexural psoriasis is common while eruptive guttate disease is rare. Methotrexate is the treatment of choice.

Leg Ulcers

Mostly are due to venous hypertension though arterial disease may be responsible in some of the cases.

MULTIPLE CHOICE QUESTIONS

1. An infant with multiple blue subcutaneous nodules ("Blueberry muffin" baby) would most likely have:
A. Congenital leukemia
B. Carcinoid from lung
C. Carcinoid of gut origin
D. None of the above

2. A 5-year-old male child has multiple hyperpigmented macules over the trunk. On rubbing the lesion with the rounded end of a pen, he developed urticarial wheal, confined to the border of the lesion. The most likely diagnosis is:
A. Fixed drug eruption
B. Lichen planus
C. Urticaria pigmentosa
D. Urticarial vasculitis

3. 'Cassals necklace' is a feature of:
A. Acrodermatitis enteropathica
B. Niacin deficiency
C. Ceruloplasmin deficiency
D. Essential fatty acid toxicity

4. Langer's lines are seen in:
A. Lichen planus
B. Atopic dermatitis
C. Psoriasis
D. Normal persons

5. Naevus depigmentosus all true *except:*
A. Usually presents in second year of life
B. Lesions may be multiple
C. Lesions may be in dermatomal or whorled pattern
D. Defect in transfer of melanosomes to keratniocytes has been postulated

6. All true of berloque dermatitis *except*:
A. Caused by buergot oil contained in perfumes
B. Wavelengths between 290-320 nn are involved
C. Deep brown pigmentation along the trickling of perfume
D. The pigmentation fades after weeks or months

7. Treatment of choice for facial port- wine stain:
A. Argon laser
B. Tunable pulsed dye laser
C. Nd-YAG laser
D. Ruby laser

8. The following disease are aggravated by exposure to sunlight *except*:
A. Freckles
B. Melanocytic naevus
C. Xeroderma pigmentosum
D. Discoid lupus erythematosus

9. Lupus perino is seen in:
A. Porphyria
B. Sarcoidosis
C. Tuberous sclerosis
D. Pellagra

10. Internal malignancy is/are frequently associated with:
A. Erythema gyratum repens
B. Erythema chronicum migrans
C. Erythema annulare centrifugum
D. All of the above

1 A 2 C 3 B 4 D 5 B 6 D 7 B 8 B 9 B 10 D

11. Acanthosis nigricans is indicative of:
A. Internal malignancy
B. Endocrine disorder
C. Blooms syndrome
D. Pigmentation of face, neck etc.
E. All of the above

12. Pruritus of renal disease:
A. Psychogenic
B. Indicates probable renal malignancy
C. Related to level of azotemia
D. Occurs in chronic pyelonephritis and chronic glomerulonephritis but not in acute nephritis

13. The following are correct statements concerning steroids used topically:
A. Halogenation decreases topical activity
B. Thinning of epidermis may occur
C. Thinning of dermis may occur
D. Systemic side-effects commonly occur
E. The rate of epidermal turnover is increased

14. Progressive pigmented purpuric dermatosis is also called:
A. Sweet syndrome
B. Darier's disease
C. Hailey-Hailey disease
D. Schamberg's disease

15. Necrobiosis lipoidica diabeticorum is most marked on:
A. Forearms B. Face
C. Front of legs D. Back of legs

16. Poor prognostic indicators for vitiligo are all *except*:
A. Long duration
B. Young age of onset
C. Leukotrichia
D. Acrofacial vitiligo

17. Half and half nails are seen in:
A. Liver disease
B. Chronic renal failure
C. COPD
D. SLE

18. All of the following diseases frequently involve both the kidney and skin *except*:
A. Polyarteritis nodosum
B. Wegner's granulomatosis
C. Erythema nodosum
D. Henoch-Schönlein purpura

19. First line treatment of keloid is:
A. Wide excision
B. Intralesional corticosteroids
C. Radiotherapy
D. Local steroids

20. Poliosis is:
A. Localised patch of white hair
B. Skin changes in poliomyelitis
C. Premature greying of hair
D. Localised patch of baldness

21. Which laser is colored blue green?
A. Argon B. CO_2
C. Ruby D. YAG

22. Which laser is selectively absorbed?
A. Argon B. CO_2
C. Ruby D. YAG

23. True about Kveim's test is:
A. Subcutaneous test
B. Highly specific for sarcoidosis
C. Dextrose extract from sarcoid tissue used
D. Has some degree of prognostic value

24. Berloque dermatitis is due to contact with:
A. Metals
B. Dyes
C. Food
D. Photosensitizing agents

11 E 12 C 13 B,C 14 D 15 C 16 B 17 A,B 18 C 19 B 20 A 21 A
22 C 23 D 24 D

25. De Morgan's spots most often require:
A. Local keratolytic agents
B. Local steroids
C. Local retinoids
D. No treatment

26. All are proposed etiological hypothesis for vitiligo *except*:
A. Autoimmune
B. Self-destruct
C. Neurogenic
D. Composite
E. Psychogenic

27. Following conditions have increased association with vitiligo *except:*
A. Thyroiditis
B. Pernicious anaemia
C. Hepatitis
D. Morphea
E. Diabetes

28. The following is true of Meirowsky phenomenon *except*:
A. Best observed in hyperpigmented skin
B. Most effective induced by UVA
C. It is a delayed tanning reaction
D. It is transient

29. All true about albinism *except*:
A. Most forms are autosomal recessive
B. Defect in enzyme tyrosinase
C. Melanocytes are completely absent in the skin
D. Melanocytes are normal in number but the melanocytes synthesize inadequate amounts of melanin
E. Depigmented or hypopigmented skin and hair, nystagmus, photophobia and decreased visual activity

30. Piebaldism—all true *except*:
A. Depigmented patches of skin present at birth
B. White forelock
C. Islands of normal or hypermelanotic skin occur in the white areas
D. Autosomal recessive inheritance

31. The primary event causing Kyrle's disease is:
A. Perforation of the epidermis
B. Abnormally fast keratinization
C. Increased rate of cell proliferation
D. All of the above

32. Malignant acanthosis nigricans is most commonly caused by:
A. Lymphoma
B. Squamous cell carcinoma
C. Adenocarcinoma
D. Mycosis fungoides

33. Pseudocanthosis Nigricans is seen in:
A. Endocrine disorders
B. Metabolic disorders
C. Abdominal cancers
D. Obese

34. Sutton's naevus is usually a benign melanocytic naevus but may be a:
A. Neuroid naevus
B. Blue naevus
C. Neuro fibroma
D. Primary or secondary malignant melanoma
E. All of the above

35. Chemicals like monebenzyle ether of hydroquinone cause skin depigmentation by:
A. Inhibiting tyrosinase
B. Destroying melanocytes
C. Preventing transfer of melanosomes
D. Decreasing melanin synthesis

25 D 26 E 27 C 28 C 29 C 30 D 31 B 32 C 33 D 34 E 35 B

36. **Cafe-au-lait macules (CALM) are associated with all *except*:**
   - A. Neurofibromatosis
   - B. McCune-Albright syndrome
   - C. Fanconi's syndrome
   - D. Acropigmentation of kitamura

37. **All modalities are used to treat vitiligo *except*:**
   - A. PUVA therapy
   - B. Potent topical steroids
   - C. Punch grafting
   - D. Tattooing
   - E. Laser

38. **The wavelength of light responsible for most cases of polymorphic light sensitive eruption is:**
   - A. 290-350 nm
   - B. 320-380 nm
   - C. 400-700 nm
   - D. 700-800 nm

39. **Erythema ab igne is caused by:**
   - A. Repeated friction
   - B. Repeated and prolonged exposure to heat
   - C. Repeated and prolonged exposure to cold
   - D. Prolonged exposure to sunlight

40. **The concentration of hydroquinone for treating chloasma should be:**
   - A. Less than 1%
   - B. 1-2%
   - C. 2-5 %
   - D. 10%

41. **Lichen spinulosus is least common on:**
   - A. Abdomen
   - B. Buttocks
   - C. Legs
   - D. Arms

42. **Blue naevus is most common on:**
   - A. Arms
   - B. Chest
   - C. Face
   - D. Legs

36 D 37 E 38 A 39 B 40 C 41 D 42 C

Chapter 20

HIV Dermatoses

Human immunodeficiency virus (HIV), the causative agent of acquired immunodeficiency syndrome (AIDS) is a retrovirus which contains single stranded RNA. HIV includes two subtypes type 1 and type 2. HIV-1 is more common in Western countries while HIV-2 in more common is South East Asia and Africa.

Mode of transmission: Principal modes of transmission are blood and blood products, sexual contact, intravenous drug abuse and passage from mother to child.

Classification: The clinical picture may be divided into:

1. Acute retroviral syndrome.
2. Asymptomatic stage.
3. Early symptomatic.
4. Late symptomatic.
5. Advanced stage.

Natural Course

Within 3-6 weeks of infection patient develops acute retroviral syndrome which is an infectious mononucleosis like illness which subsides by itself and the person remains asymptomatic for quite some time ranging from 3-20 years. After which the immune status decreases and viral load increases, producing various opportunistic infections, neoplasias and other symptoms.

Disorders associated with or indicative of AIDS are:

- Persistent generalized lymphadenopathy.
- Constitutional symptoms (fever 101.3°F, diarrhoea > 1 month).
- Idiopathic thrombocytopenic purpura.
- Peripheral neuropathy.
- Pelvic inflammatory disease.
- Listeriosis.
- Oral hairy leucoplakia.
- Cervical squamous intraepithelial lesion.
- HIV encephalopathy.
- Progressive multifocal encephalopathy.
- Mycobacterium tuberculosis infection.
- Mycobacterium avium intracellulare infection.
- Pneumonia: Recurrent with > 2 episodes in 12 months.
- Candidiasis esophageal, pulmonary.
- Cryptococcosis.
- Coccidiodomycosis.
- Histoplasmosis.
- Pneumocystis carinii pneumonia.
- Kaposi sarcoma.
- Toxoplasmosis.
- Cervical cancer.

Mucocutaneous disorders indicative of HIV:

a. **Highly indicative of HIV infection**—Exanthem of acute retroviral syndrome, proximal subungual orychomycosis, chronic herpetic ulcers, oral hairy leukoplakia, kaposis sarcoma, eosinophilic folliculitis and mutliple facial molluscum contagiosum.

b. **Strongly associated with HIV infection**—Any sexually transmitted disease, herpes zoster, signs of injected drug use and candidiasis either oropharyngeal or recurrent vulvovaginal.

c. **May be associated with HIV infection**—Generalized lymphadenopathy, seborrheic dermatitis (extensive, refractory to therapy) and apthous ulcers (recurrent, refractory to therapy).

Diagnosis of HIV infection can be made by antibody detection, antigen detection or virus detection.

a. **Anti body detection** can be carried out by:
   1. Enzyme linked immunosorbent assay (ELISA).
   2. Immunoblot (Western blot).
   3. Indirect immunofluorescence (IFA) test.
   4. Latex agglutination test, and
   5. Solid surface dot-blot enzyme immunoassay.

b. **Antigen detection** can be done by:
   P24 antigen assay, and
   Polymerase chain reaction (PCR).

c. **Virus detection**
   1. *Culture:* Out of the above said tests ELISA is commonly used as screening test and P24 antigen assay is used for detecting infection in window period also Western blot, IFA and PCR are used as confirmatory tests.

Treatment

Treatment of opportunistic infections and good nutritious diet are as important as for other diseases and specific therapy is as follows:

1. **Nucleoside analogues**—Zidovudine (AZT), Lamivudine (3TC), Didanosine (ddI), Zalcitabine (ddC) and Stavundine (d4T) are available.
2. **Non-nucleoside reverse transcriptase inhibitor**—Nevirapine, Delaviridine (DLV) and Efavirenz are available.
3. **Protease inhibitors**—Saquinavir, Indinavir, Ritonavir, Nelfinavir and Amprenavir can be used.

MULTIPLE CHOICE QUESTIONS

1. All true of oral hairy leukoplakia *except*:
A. Usually asymptomatis
B. Proliferation of Ebstein-Barr virus in the epithelium is thought to be responsible
C. Candidiasis may co-exist
D. Treatment with acyclovir should be instituted in all cases without delay
E. Characterized by vertically ribbed keratinized plaques along lateral borders of the tongue

2. All true of syphilis co-existing with HIV infection *except*:
A. Syphilis probably increases transmissibility of HIV
B. Seroconversion of syphilis in HIV is same as in HIV negative patients
C. A severe form of syphilis with necrotizing lesions may be seen
D. There is relatively rapid progression to tertiary syphilis and neurosyphilis

3. All of the following are highly indicative of HIV infection *except*:
A. Oral hairy leukoplakia
B. Kaposi's sarcoma
C. Multiple molluscum contagiosum lesion on face of adult
D. Recurrent herpes labialis

4. AIDS is caused by:
A. HTLV-1 B. HTLV-2
C. HTLV-3 D. HTLV-4

5. Following drug is contraindicated in HIV patients:
A. Rifampicin B. Cotrimoxazole
C. Penicillins D. Thiacetazone

6. All are cutaneous manifestations of AIDS *except*:
A. Kaposis sarcoma
B. Oral hairy leukoplakia
C. Seborrheic dermatitis
D. Melanoma

1 D 2 B 3 D 4 C 5 D 6 D

Chapter 21

Disorders of Sebaceous Eccrine & Apocrine Glands

DISORDERS OF THE SEBACEOUS GLANDS

Acne Vulgaris

Acne vulgaris is a self limited disease, seen frequently in adolescents, primarily involves the sebaceous follicles. Most cases of acne are pleomorphic, presenting with a variety of lesions—comedones, papules, pustules, nodules, and as sequelae to active lesions—pitted or hypertrophic scars.

PATHOGENESIS

Four major factors are involved in the pathogenesis:

1. Increased sebum production.
2. Hypercornification of the pilosebaceous duct.
3. Microbial flora.
4. Inflammation.

Increased Sebum Production

Acne patients, male and female, excrete on average more sebum than normal subjects and the level of secretion correlates with the acne severity.

Ductal Hypercornification

Hypercornification of pilosebaceous ducts presents histologically as microcomedones and clinically as blackheads and whiteheads. Thus comedones represent the retention of hyperproliferating ductal keratinocytes in the duct.

Bacteria

Acne is not infectious. However three major organisms isolated—Propionibacteria (P. acnes, P. granulosum, P. avidum), Staphylococcus epidermidis and Malassezia furfur. Environment of bacteria (i.e. low pH, reduced oxygen tension and bacterial lipases, proteases etc.) more important than absolute numbers.

Inflammation

The dermal inflammation is not caused by bacteria in the dermis but from inflammatory mediators that diffuse from the follicle where they are produced by P. acnes.

Treatment

Treatment involves counselling, acne assessment and appropriate and ethical prescribing based on the history, acne severity, lesion type and the psychological effects of the disease. The various modalities of treatment can be classified into topical and systemic therapies.

Topical

- *Predominantly comedolytic:*
  1. Tretinoin (reduce number of existing comedones and prevent formation of new comedones by loosening ductal keratinocytes).

2. Adapalene.
3. Azelaic acid.

- *Predominantly antimicrobial:*
  1. Clindamycin.
  2. Erythromycin.
  3. Benzoyl peroxide.
  4. Tetracycline.
  5. Predominantly anti-inflammatory.
  6. Adapalene.
  7. Topical antibiotics.
  8. Combination preparations.
  9. Zinc and erythromycin.
  10. Benzoyl peroxide and erythromycin.

Systemic

- Oral antibiotics (Oral minocycline, doxycycline, erythromycin trimethoprim).
- Hormones (anti-andrognes like cyproterone acetate, flutamide, estrogens, spironolactone, finasteride).
- Isotretinoin.
- Corticosteroids (co-prescribed with isotretinion in severe acne variants).
  - *DOC*—Isotretinoin–0.5-1.0 mg/kg a day.
  - *Optimium dose*—120-160 mg/kg CUMULATIVE.

Disorders of Eccrine Sweat Glands

Disorders of eccrine sweat glands may be broadly classified into four—chromhidrosis, hyperhidrosis, hypo-or anhidrosis and miliaria.

Chromhidrosis: It means secretion of coloured sweat.

Hyperhidrosis: It means excessive sweating which could be localized or generalized. It may occur in consequence of a number of causes. Most commonly excessive sweating of the palms and soles occurs during mental stress, and may be associated with tachycardia and vasomotor instability.

Tap water iontophoresis is the most effective, safe and inexpensive therapeutic modality for palmoplantar hyperhidrosis. Local injection of botulinum toxin is a new modality of treatment for palmar hyperhidrosis.

Disorders of Apocrine Glands

FOX-FORDYCE—Itchy papules on axilla.

MULTIPLE CHOICE QUESTIONS

1. **For dyce pots are:**
   A. Ectopic apocrine glands found in axilla
   B. Ectopic sebaceous glands
   C. Seen in vitamin A deficiency
   D. Another name for freckles

2. **A young female presents with erythema, increasing on exposure to sunlight along with papulo-pustules, telangiectasia over both cheeks and a bullous nose—likely diagnosis:**
   A. SLE B. Sarcoidosis
   C. Photosensitivity D. Rosacea

3. **Treatment of choice for severe nodulocystic acne:**
   A. Doxycycline
   B. Oral retinoids
   C. Minocycline
   D. Topical retinoids

4. **Hidradenitis suppurativa is a disease of:**
   A. Apocrine glands
   B. Eccrine glands
   C. Sebaceous glands
   D. Apo-eccrine glands

5. **Bromhidrosis is usually confined to:**
   A. Axillae B. Genitalia
   C. Feet D. Nape of neck

6. **The following may be used in acne vulgaris *except*:**
   A. Mometasone
   B. Topical erythromycin
   C. Tretinoin
   D. Benozyl peroxide

7. **Steroid acne is more common in:**
   A. Face
   B. Hands
   C. Legs
   D. Trunk

8. **Oral retinoid is indicated in the treatment of:**
   A. Severe acne vulgaris
   B. Pemphigus vulgaris
   C. Lupus vulgaris
   D. Erythema multiforme

9. **Hidradenitis suppurativa is a disease of :**
   A. Apocrine glands
   B. Eccrine glands
   C. Apo-eccrine glands
   D. Sebaceous glands

10. **Steatocystoma multiplex is most common on:**
    A. Genitalia B. Legs
    C. Chest D. Face

11. **Following are effects of benzoyl peroxide *except*:**
    A. Potent oxidizing property
    B. Sebosuppressant
    C. Melanocyte stimulation
    D. Comedolytic

12. **Milium is most common on:**
    A. Face B. Chest
    C. Legs D. Genitalia

13. **Hydrocystoma is most common on:**
    A. Arms B. Legs
    C. Chest D. Face

---

1 B 2 D 3 B 4 A 5 A,C 6 A 7 A,D 8 D 9 C 10 B 11 C
12 A 13 D

14. Richner-Hanhart syndrome is associated with all of the following *except*:
A. A deficiency of hepatic cytosolic tyrosine aminotransferase
B. Painful keratoderma
C. Photophobia
D. Reversal of the skin lesions as well as eye lesions with early dietary intervention with a high tyrosine and high phenylalanine diet

15. Seborrheic dermatitis is more successfully treated with:
A. A surgery
B. Topical steroids
C. Radiation
D. Abrasives

16. Treatment of acne vulgaris may include all *except:*
A. Cryotherapy
B. Oestrogens
C. UV light
D. Androgens

17. Which of the following type of lesion of acne is common in infants and young children?
A. Papule B. Pustule
C. Comedone D. Nodule

18. Bromhidrosis may be produced by intake of the following *except:*
A. Asfoetida B. Ginger
C. Onions D. Garlic

14 D 15 B 16 D 17 C 18 B

Chapter 22

Paediatric Dermatology

Some skin disorders are transient in newborn but make the parents nervous and anxious about their outcome, while other skin disorders develop later on during infancy dermatitis or childhood. Some of these disorders are exclusive to children (Cradle cap, napkin dermatitis, acrodermatitis enteropathica, primary herpetic gingivostomatitis) while others are common in children (Pediculosis capitis, scabies, molluscum contagiosum, warts, chicken pox, tinea capitis, atopic dermatitis, oral thrush, Henoch-Schönlein purpura, acute hemorrhagic edema of infancy and popular urticaria).

Transient Cutaneous Lesions in Newborn

- Vernix caseosa—golden yellow staining of vernix caseosa occur in haemolytic disease of the newborn and post maturity.
- Acrocyanosis—cyanosis seen in acral areas in a neonate.
- Erythema neonatorum—within a few hours of birth—erythema fades spontaneously within 24-48 hours.
- Harlequin colour change—upper half of the body becoming pale and the lower half a deep red colour, with a sharp midline demarcation between the two, stay for half a minute to 20 minutes, in a full term or pattern newborn seen during first week of life.
- Cutis marmorata—this marbling change due to reticular blue vascular pattern seen in infancy.
- Physiological scaling of the newborn seen in upto 75% of the normal neonates.
- Sebaceous gland hyperplasia characterized by multiple, uniform, pin point yellowish papules, most prominent on the nose, cheeks, upper lip and forehead, but may be visible on the upper trunk, especially the areolae, genitalia and the limbs. This phenomenon is associated with milia which represents minute follicular epidermal cysts.
- Linea alba becomes pigmented in about 8% of babies.
- Exaggerated pigmentation of the scrotum occurs in about 30% of oriental neonates, generally associated with Mongolian spots.
- Milia represent miniature epidermal inclusion cysts that originate from sebaceous apparatus of vellus hair. Epstein pearls are clinically and histologically the intra oral counterpart of facial milia.
- Succulent gums (Sucking pads)—a whitish hue to the oral mucosa.
- Erythema toxicum neonatourm (Toxic erythema of the new born, etythema neonatorum) presents as asymptomatic macular erythema on the trunk within first 48 hours of birth. Subsequently, it may evolve into urticarial papules

of pustules. Recovery occurs in 3 days. Smears of the pustule contents demonstrate inflammatory cells, more than 90% of which are eosinophilis. There is an associated blood eosinophilia in 50% cases.

- Mongolian spots—are blue gray pigmentation areas presents at birth on the sacral area of the normal infants in dark skinned races. Edwin Baez, thinking this a characteristic of Mongolian race, named it as Mongolian spot. The Chinese people believed that the mark is the imprint of their "God of birth". As the child is born, the God gives it as a 'spank' or 'kick' to give it start in life, whereas the Japanese believed that the spot was the consequence of coitus performed during pregnancy. It usually disappears during the first decade and in small percentage (3-4%) persist beyond this into adult life.
- Acne neonatorum (Neonatal acne)—develops with the first 30 days of life.
- Perianal dermatitis is an erythema centered on the anus, occasionally accompanied by erosion and bleeding at 4th to 7th day of life.
- Transient neonatal pustulosis (Transient neonatal pustular melanosis) invariably presents at birth. It is characterized by the presence of fragile superficial pustules mainly over the chin, neck, forehead, back and buttock. Hyperpigmented macules develop subsequently. They may persist for 3 months and affected infants are otherwise normal. Pustules are formed due to subcorneal collection of neutrophilis with a few eosinophils, Bacterial culture is negative. Pigmented macules demonstrate basal and supra basal increase in pigmentation only, apparently without pigmentary incontinence.

Skin Disorders in Children (Paediatric Dermatoses)

Skin disorders are extremely common in our population and approximately 6% of visits to all physicians entail a problem of the skin, hair or nails. However, dermatologists see only approximately 40% of these patients. Dermatological problems manifesting as primary secondary cutaneous complaints, constitute at least 30% of all outpatient visits to a pediatrician and 30% of all visits to dermatologists involve patients of pediatric age group.

The vast majority of complaints related to the skin in children can be easily recognized and treated by non-specialist. Those common diseases have been classified in the Table 22.1.

Table 22.1: Classification of common paediatric dermatoses

1. Infestations and infections
   a. Parasitic infestations—Pediculosis capitis, scabies
   b. Bacterial infections—Pyodermas
   c. Viral infections—Molluscum contagiosum, warts, herpes simplex, chicken pox, herpes zoster
   d. Fungal infections—Tinea capitis, tinea corporis, piryriasis versicolor, candidiasis
2. Dermatitis and eczema—Infantile seborrheic dermatitis, diaper or napkin dermatitis, atopic dermatitis, infective dermatitis
3. Urticaria
4. Exanthems—Viral exanthems (Measles, rubella, roseola infantum, erythema infectiosum)
5. Drug eruptions
6. Pigmentary disorders—Postinflammatory pigmentation, hypopigmentary disorders (Pityriasis alba, vitiligo, nervus achromicus, ash leaf macule, albinism), hyperpigmentary disorders (Mongolian spots, café au lait macules)
7. Disease of hair and nails—Tinea capitis, alopecia areata, diffuse alopecia, twenty nail dystrophy
8. Genetic disease of the skin—Ichthyosis, acrodermatitis enteropathica
9. Collagen vascular diseases—Connective tissue diseases (Lupus erythematosus, scleroderma and dermatomyositis) and vasculitic syndrome (Henoch-Schönlein purpura, acute hemorrhagic edema of infancy and polyteritis nodosa)
10. Miscellaneous conditions—Papular urticaria, miliaria, miliaria cystalina, psoriasis, hemangiomas, chilblains

Some Important Viral Exanthems in Children Measles (Rubeola, Morbilli)

- The term measles is thought to come from Latin "misellus" or "misella", a diminutive of Latin "miser" meaning miserable.

- It is caused by measles virus (a paramyxovirus, RNA virus).
- Incubation period is 10-11 days.
- Measles is a universal highly contagious disease of children. It has a characteristic prodrome of 3-4 days that consists of **high fever, cough, coryza, a striking palpebral conjunctivitis with photophobia and Koplik's spots, which precede the apperance of florid generalized macular and papular rash.**
- The first lesion to appear on the soft palate as blochy erythema, but the most appear as tiny white lesions surrounded by an erythematous ring (grain of sands).
- Koplik's spots precedes the onset of generalized rash by 1-2 days, remain for two to three days and are usually heavily clustered on the mucosa opposite the second molar.
- The purplish red rash on the body **appears first behind the ears** and over the forehead, and then spreads slowly to involve the entire body by third day. The eruption extends downwards over the neck, shoulders and trunk and then distally over the upper and lower extremities.
- Uncomplicated measles runs a self-limited course lasting about 10 days.
- There is no specific therapy for measles.

Rubella (German Measles)

- Rubella virus is a togavirus, commonly recovered from pharynx.
- Incubation periods is **14-21 days**.
- Rubella is a common communicable infection of children and young adults characterized by **a short prodromal period; enlargement of cervical, suboccipital and postauricular glands and a rash of approximately 2 to 3 days duration.**
- An exanthem **Forschheimer's sign** is present in upto 20% of patients during the prodromal period or on the first day of the rash. Dull-red macules or petechiae are confined to the soft palate.
- The disease has rare sequelae apart from devastating effect on the fetus.

Exanthem Subitum (Sixth Disease, Roseola Infantum)

- Caused by human herpes virus type 6 (DNA virus).
- Incubation period is 10-15 days.
- Most common exanthema with fever in children under age group of 2 years.
- Prodromal fever is usually high. Fever drops on fourth day.
- Convulsions and lymphadenopathy may accompany it.
- Clinically, a morbilliform erythema consisting of rose coloured discrete macules appears on the neck, trunk and buttocks.
- Often there is a blanched halo around the lesions.
- The lesions resolve in 1 to 2 days.
- Other common associated findings include otitis media, diarrhoea and meningoencephalitis.
- In adults HHV—6 infection resembles otitis mononucleosis.
- Treatment—acyclovir, ganciclovir.

Erythema Infectiosum (Fifth Disease)

- Exanthematous disease occurring in patients with primary human parvo virus B_{19} infection (DNA virus).
- Incubation period is **4-14 days.**
- More commonly seen in school children.
- Infection is spread by respiratory droplets during the prodrome.
- Constitutional symptoms are absent or very minimal.
- **"Slapped cheek" appearance** (1 to 4 days).
- Erythematous popular eruption over the upper and lower extremites spreading to trunk. Assumes a lacelike or reticulated appearance as it fades.

- Recurrent evanescent stage (for weeks or months) is performed seen in older children and adolescent.
- Adults may present with atypical rash and arthritis.
- Complication—Hydrops foetails (maternal infection) and aplastic crisis.
- Treatment—supportive.

Gianotti-Crosti Syndrome

- Infantile popular acrodermatitis, or the Gianotti-Crosti syndrome, presents with symmetric erythematous lichenoid papules on the face, extremities and buttocks, usually sparing the trunk.
- The eruption is not pruritic and may be accompanied by splenomegaly, hepatitis and lymphadenopathy.
- The process often occurs in young children after an upper respiratory tract illness.
- Pathologic specimens show a perivascular infiltration of lymphocytes and histiocytes in the upper portion of the dermis.
- While the syndrome has been associated with hepatitis B and enterovirus infection, several cases have been associated with acute EBV infection.

- While the syndrome has been associated with hepatitis B and enterovirus infection, several cases have been associated with acute EBV infection.

Some Other Important Entities

Henoch-Schönlein Purpura

- Henoch-Schönlein purpura is an IgA mediated vasculitis syndrome affecting skin, joints, GIT and kidneys.
- It usually occurs below the age of 20 years.
- The eruption may begin as crops of palpable purpuric lesions or urticarial rash in the lower legs and buttock.
- Abdominal symptoms such as colic, vomiting and diarrhea are seen in two-third of the patients.
- Polyarthralgia is seen in most patients and renal involvement can rarely lead to chronic nephritis.
- *Diagnosis:* Histopathology shows leucocytoclastic vasculitis and immunofluorescence demonstrates IgA deposition around blood vessels.
- *Treatment:* No specific treatment available. Antibiotics and corticosteroids can be given to alleviate symptoms.

Urticaria Pigmentosa

Urticaria pigmentosa is the most common type of cutaneous mastocytosis that occurs due to the accumulation of mast cells in the skin:

- The skin lesions are itchy small, yellow tan to reddish brown macules scattered all over the body.
- Mild trauma such as scratching or rubbing the lesions may cause urtication and erythema around macules this is **known as Darier's sign.**
- Urticaria pigmentosa is associated with Pruritus which may be exacerbated by temperature, friction, spicy food, alcohol and drugs.
- *Diagnosis:* Histopathlogy shows mast cell infiltration in the dermis.
- *Treatment:* Avoidance of precipitating factors and antihistaminics.

Langerhans Cell Histiocytosis (LCH)

Langerhans cell histiocytosis a disease that results due to the proliferation or cells like Langerhans cells called as LCH cell (share the ultrastructural features with Langerhans cells—containing Birbeck granules) in any organ. This "LCH cell" is about four to five times larger than small lymphocytes; has an irregular and vesiculated nucleus; is often reniform (kidney shaped); and has abundant, slightly consinophilic cytoplasm.

- It is broadly classified into entities such as Letterer-Siwe disease, Hand-Schuller Christian disease and eosinophilic granuloma
- **Eosinophilic granuloma** occurs due to localized proliferation of "LCH cells" in the bones, skin, lymph nodes, lung, liver and spleen.
- **Hand-Schuller Christian syndrome** is a chronic multisystemic disease known by the triad of exophthalmos, multiple skull lesions and diabetes insipidus **Letterer-Siwe disease** is usually seen in children less than 1 year. It is characterized by seborrheic dermatitis like rash with hemorrhagic popular, vesicular, pustular and ulcerated lesions in the intertriginous regions and trunk.
- Letterer-Siwe disease is often associated with hepatosplenomegaly, dysfunction of liver, lungs hematopoietic system. Lytic lesions may be seen in skull bones.
- *Diagnosis:* Histopathology shows LCH cell infiltration of the lesions.
- *Treatment:* Localized forms can be treated with intralesional steroids or surgery. Multisystemic involvement needs chemotherapy.

MULTIPLE CHOICE QUESTIONS

1. **An infant presents with hoarseness of voice and waxy papules on face and eyelids, probable diagnosis is:**
   A. Mucinosis
   B. Amyloidosis
   C. Lipoid proteinosis
   D. Fabry's disease
2. **"Creeping eruption" is caused due to larvae of:**
   A. *Ankylostomacaninum*
   B. Strongyloides stercoralis
   C. Guinea worm
   D. Enterobius vernicularis
3. **Erythema infectiosum is caused by:**
   A. Echoviruses
   B. Paroviruses
   C. Paramyxovirus
   D. Coxsackie virus
4. **Gianotti-Crosti syndrome is often characterised by eruptions on extremities and face:**
   A. Macular
   B. Papular
   C. Vesicular
   D. Bullous
5. **Vogt-Koyanagi-Harada syndrome comprises:**
   A. Involvement of brain and meninges
   B. Bilateral uveities, labyrinthitis and deafness
   C. Poliosis, leucoderma, alopecia
   D. All of the above
   E. None of the above
6. **Incontinentia pigmenti is characterized by all *except*:**
   A. Vesiculobullous lesions
   B. Hyperpigmentation
   C. Telangiectases
   D. Verrucous lesions
   E. Hypopigmentation
7. **A localized area of cutis verticis gyrata in a newborn is most likely to be:**
   A. A glioma
   B. A meningioma
   C. Caput succedaneum
   D. Cutis laxa
   E. A naevoid tumour
8. **A 2-year-old child with an upper respiratory infection suddenly develops a bluish red ill defined warm oedematous plaque on face. This picture is typical of:**
   A. Erysipelas
   B. Anthrax
   C. Disseminated intravascular coagulation
   D. Haemophilus influenzae cellulitis
9. **Erythema toxicum in a neonate indicates:**
   A. Staphylococcal sepsis
   B. Pneumococcimia
   C. Drug hypersensitivity
   D. Is not of any significance

1 C 2 A 3 B 4 B 5 D 6 C 7 E 8 D 9 D

10. Regarding hemangiomas, the following are true:

A. Salmon patch disappears after the age of one
B. Portwine stain present throughout life
C. Strawberry haemangioma disappears on its own, usually by 7 years of age
D. All are correct

11. A 10-year-old child complaining of pustular lesions for 1 year duration shows dark crusted lesions and superficial scars on legs. The most likely diagnosis is:

A. Impetigo contagiosa
B. Bockhart's impetigo
C. Tropical sores
D. Ecthyma

10 D 11 D

Chapter 23

Dermatological Therapy

TOPICAL THERAPY

Successful dermatologic therapy depends both upon the active drug and the physical properties of the formulation. The choice of vehicle, the frequency and quantity of application and the appropriateness of these factors for the skin often determine the efficacy and tolerability of topical therapy. Choosing the right drug and the right vehicle is of paramount importance.

The spectrum of inflammation with corresponding range of appropriate dermatologic vehicles.

Acute inflammation: Wet dressings (water) erythema, edema, vesiculation, oozing, powders, lotions, aerosols, sprays crusting, infection, pruritus.

Cream (Oil in water emulsions) Gels

Chronic inflammation-erythema, ointments (Water in oil, inert bases) scaling, lichenification, dryness, pruritus.

CLASSIFICATION AND CLINICAL APPLICATION OF TOPICAL FORMULATIONS

The term vehicle is used for that substances that bring specific drugs into contact with the skin. The vehicle itself may be beneficial by producing cooling, protective, emollient, occlusive or astringent properties. Ideally they are non-toxic, stable and do not sensitize with repeated use. These vehicles may have an effect on the skin or epithelial metabolism. Petrolatum for example: interferes with the oxidation of arachidonic acid and inhibit synthesis of prostaglandins in animal skin. It also retards the rate of epidermal healing, whereas creams and lotions increase this rate. For any drug to be effective topically, it must be formulated at the proper concentration and in the proper vehicle.

The most important vehicles can be divided into monophasic, biphasic and triphasic forms.

Powders: These are used for cosmetic and hygienic purposes. Powders decrease friction and increase surface area thereby have a soothing, cooling and anti-pruritic effect. These should not be used in flexures with weeping skin as abrasive clumps would be formed. Talc (anhydrous magnesium silicate) might lead to granulomatous reaction in wounds. Tolnaftate and nystatin have anti-fungal properties.

Wet Dressings: These are indicated in acute inflammatory conditions, erosions, ulcers and bullous diseases. These have cooling and drying effect, cause vasoconstriction and cleanse the skin of exudates, crusts and debris. Burrows' solution (Aluminium acetate) and condy's compresses ($KMnO_4$) are the commonly used wet dressings in dermatological practice.

Baths: These are useful in delivering medication in widespread less exudative eruptions and to cleanse the skin of adherent scales and debris.

But these cause maceration hence duration of immersion to be limited to thirty minutes. Soothing and antipruritic colloid additives like oatmeal and starch can be added.

Tinctures: Tinctures are alcoholic or hydroalcoholic solutions. These agents have mostly gone into disrepute due to their staining and irritant properties.

Solutions: Solvents in which active ingredients are dissolved to clarity.

Lotions: These are liquid preparations in which inert or active medications are suspended or dissolved. They are well suited for use in hairy and intertriginous regions as they are easy to apply and to do not predispose to folliculitis.

Calamine lotion (ZnO_2 + 0.5% $Fe_2 O_3$) is a commonly used example which has anti-pruritic, bland and soothing agent.

Gels: These are solution of solvents such as water, acetone, alcohol or prophylene alcohol thickened with organic polymers such as carbopols. Gels are appropriate for use on hairy areas and cosmetically acceptable but lack any protective or emollient properties.

Greasy Bases: The principle use of oil is the removal of fat miscible applications from skin oils added to baths may function as emollients.

BIPHASIC VEHICLES

Shake lotions: These are solid in liquid lotions that require shaking before use.

Creams: These are emulsions of oil. These are more lubricating than creams and have a better topical penetration. Petrolatum, lanolin, euccerin, nivea oil and silicone ointments are the example of commonly used ointments.

Pastes: Pastes are ointments into which 20-50% powder (e.g. ZnO_2, starch) is incorporated. These are used in the treatment of ulcers, chronic exudative dermatoses and thick, lichenified plaques. Lassar's paste (stiff paste of ZnO_2, cornstarch and white petrolatum) is used in treatment of psoriasis.

Emollients: These are occlusive agents which increase hydration of stratum corneum and hence make skin soft and pliable. Petrolatum, mineral oil and baby oil are the most effective but least cosmetically acceptable.

Humectants: These are hygroscopic agents which draw moisture into the skin.

APPLICATION AND DOSAGE OF TOPICAL THERAPY

Amount of topical medication needed for single application:

- Area treated one application (g).
- Hands, head, face, anogenital area 2.
- One arm, anterior or posterior trunk 3.
- One leg 4.
- Entire body 30-60.

Finger tip unit (FTU) is a practical and simple means of explaining how much ointment is adequate to cover a specific region IFTU is the amount of ointment expressed from a tube with 5 mm diameter nozzle applied from the distal skin crease to the tip of index finger.

1 FTm = .5 g

TOPICAL CORTICOSTEROIDS

Topical steroids are the most frequently used drugs in Dermatology O.P.D.

These are classified according to the British National Formulary into 4 classes and American classification into 7 classes. Clobetasone propionate cream and ointment (0.05%) and betamethasone dipropionate cream (0.05%) in optimized vehicle have been classified as superpotent while desonide cream (0.05%), hydrocortisone and prednisolone have been classified as mild. Vasoconstrictor assays and therapeutic trials are carried out for classification according to potency. Topical steroids act by vasoconstriction, immunosuppression, anti-proliferative and anti-inflammatory actions.

Psoriasis (intertriginous), ectopic dermatitis (children), seborrheic dermatitis and intertrigo are highly responsive dermatosis while palmoplantar psoriasis, psoriasis of nails, pemphigus, granuloma annulare and sarcoidosis are not very responsive.

The adverse effects of topical steroids include epidermal and dermal atrophy, melanocyte inhibition, purpura, striae, permanent vasodilatation and in some cases systemic side-effects like growth retardation and cushingoid features may be seen intra-lesional injections near the eye may lead to blindness.

TOPICAL ANTIBIOTICS

These are commonly used in the treatment of acne, superficial infections like impetigo, leg ulcers, wound infections and post-surgical wounds. The widely used antibiotics include:

1. *Mupirocin:* It is a 2% ointment. It acts by inhibition of bacterial protein synthesis and is active against most exam positive bacteria including multiresistant staphylococcus aureus (MRSA).
2. *Neomycin and Framycetin:* These are active against aerobic gram-negative bacteria but have a very high risk of contact allergic dermatitis.
3. *Gentamycin:* Spectrum is same as neomycin but is more active against pseudomonas.
4. *Fusidic acid:* It acts by inhibiting the elongation of polypeptide chain and is active against staphylococcus, erythrasma and infected eczemas.
5. *Metronidazole:* Useful in treatment of rosacea and decubitus ulcers.
6. *Silver sulfadiazine:* This is the only sulfonamide used topically and is effective in burns and wounds.

TOPICAL ANTIVIRAL

The use of topical antiviral in dermatology is still controversial. The various topical antivirals being used include:

- *Acyclovir:* Shows maximum activity against HSV-1, but is also effective against HSV-2, VZV and EBV. The indications for use include recurrent herpes labialis, HSV-2 infections and immunocompromised persons.
- *Idoxuridine:* It is useful for HSV keratitis.
- *Podophyllin:* 25% podophyllin is effective for genital warts but it is associated with burning of surrounding skin.
- *5-Fluorouracil:* Useful for solar keratosis, superficial basal cell carcinoma, Bowen's disease and resistant vulvo-vaginal condylomas.
- *MCAA (Monochloro acetic acid):* Useful in treatment of plantar warts.

TOPICAL ANTI-FUNGALS

These are useful in treatment of superficial fungal infections like dermatophytosis, candidiasis and P. versicolor. The various topical anti-fungals being used include.

Allylamines (e.g.: Naftifine, Terbinafine).

These are fungicidal drugs which remain in skin upto 7 days. They are very effective but expensive and have the side-effects of local burning, pruritus, dryness and erythema.

AZOLES (e.g. Clotrimazole, econazole, ketoconazole, miconazole, sulconazole).

All these drugs are fungistatic ketaconazole is effective against pityriasis versicolor.

- *Ciclopiroxolamine:* It is a fungicidal and fungistatic with anti-inflammatory properties.
- *Polyenes (Nystatin):* Is active against candidiasis especially oral thrush.
- *Whitfields ointment:* This is a fungistatic and keratolytic mixture of 12% benzoic acid and 6% salicyclic acid.

KEY SYSTEMIC DRUGS

Corticosteroids

The corticosteroids bind to specific cytoplasmic receptors in the target cell and the steroid receptor complex then undergoes modification and is translocated to the nucleus effects. Their modes of actions are:

1. Anti-inflammatory.
2. Anti-allergic, and
3. Immunosuppressive.

Dosage

The intermediate acting steroids namely prednisolone is commonly used at a dose of 1 mg/kg body weight/day.

Indications

1. Autoimmune bullous dermatoses (pemhigus, buttous pemphigoid, epidermolysis bullosa acquisita, etc.).
2. Drug eruptions (erythema multiforme, Stevens Johnson syndrome, TEN).
3. Connective tissue disorders (SLE, polymyositis, dermatomyositis, progressive systemic sclerosis).
4. Severe dermatitis (atopic dermatitis, contact dermatitis, photodermatoses).
5. Neutrophilic dermatoses (pyoderma gangrenosum, Sweet's syndrome).
6. Sarcoidosis.
7. Leprosy in severe reaction.
8. Urticaria, angioedema and capillary hemangiomas.

Contraindication

There are no absolute contraindication. The relative contraindications are: Peptic ulcer disease, any focus of infection including tuberculosis, hypertension, glaucoma, cataract, hyperlipiderma, renal calculi, first trimester of pregnancy and children.

Side-Effects

1. *Metabolic disturbances:* Diabetes, faciotruncal obesity, hyperlipidermia, protein hypercatabolism, etc.
2. *Bone disturbances:* Osteoporosis, avascular necrosis of the bone, growth retardation.
3. *Muscular disorders:* Steroid myopathy, amyotrophy, tendon rupture.
4. *Cutaneous effects:* Acneiform eruptions, atrophy, telangiectasia, easy bruising, alopecia/hypertrichosis, cutaneous infection, striae distensae.
5. *Electrolyte disturbances:* Sodium retention and potassium depletion.
6. *Endocrine changes:* Inhibition of the hypothalamo-hypophyseal suprarenal axis.
7. *Infections:* Acute bacterial infection, tuberculosis, viral infection, parasitic disease.
8. *Neuropsychiatric disorders:* Neuropathy, psychosis, pseudotumour cerebri.
9. *Ocular effects:* Posterior subcapsular cataract, open angle glaucoma, aggravation of an existing infection.
10. *Gastric disturbance:* Peptic ulcer disease.
11. *Hematologic alteration:* Leucocytosis, eosinopenia and lymphopenia.

Griseofulvin

Griseofulvin is the most frequently used systemic drug in the treatment of dermatophytosis. It is a fungistatic agent derived from penicillin grisefulvum with selective activity against dermatophytes only. In addition to its antifungal activity, it is also a weak vasodilator and inhibits leucocyte chemotaxis.

Dosage

The daily recommended dose in 10 mg/kg body weight/day to a maximum of 1 gm daily, given in a single dose or in two divided doses. For ringworm of the trunk, hand or foot, it is given for a period of 4 to 6 weeks. For scalp infection 8 to 12 weeks and in nail infection for 12 to 18 months.

Side-Effects

The most commonly reported adverse effects are headache and gastrointestinal side-effects namely dyspepsia, nausea and diarrhoea. Other side-effects are photosensitivity, urticaria, erythema multiforme, maculopapular skin rash, serum sickness, angioedema and vesicular eruption. The other uncommon but serious adverse effects include hepatic and renal insufficiency, severe leukopenia, peripheral neuropathy, mental confusion and blurred vision. It can also precipitate SLE.

Acyclovir

Acyclovir is a synthetic guanosine analogue which is widely used for the treatment of herpes simplex virus and varicella zoster virus infections. Acyclovir, a prodrug, initially undergoes monphosphorylation by herpes virus encoded thymidine kinase and is activated to acyclovir triphosphate (by cellular kinase) which is the active antiviral moiety. Acyclovir is highly selective because only virus infected cells are able to phosphorylate acycloir.

Dosage

The recommended dose for the treatment of HSV infection is 200 mg 5 times a day or 400 mg three times a day for 7 to 10 days. For varicella and herpes zoster, the dose is 800 mg orally 5 times a day 7 to 10 days.

Side-Effects

They are renal crystalluria, interstitial nephritis, seizures, tremors, etc.

Antihistamines

Classification

Class I: First generation H1 type antihistamines – These traditional antihistamines are competitive blockers (reversible) and can be displaced by high levels of histamines and they dissociate from the receptors easily. They are divided into 6 groups.

1. Alkylamine—Pheniramine maleate (25-50 mg 2-3 times daily)
   - Chlopheniramine malcate (4 mg thrice daily).
2. Ethanolamine—Clemastine fumarate (1 mg twice daily)
   - Embramine hydrochloride (25-50 mg/day).
   - Bromodiphenyl hydramine hydrochloride.
   - Diphenhydramine hydrochloride (25-50 mg thrice daily), citrate.
3. Ethylenediamine—Mepyramine maleate
   - Pyrilamine maleate.
   - Tripleamine citrate, HCl.
4. Phenothiazine—Promethazine HCl (25 mg twice daily).
   - Methdilazine HCl.
5. Piperidine—Cyproheptadine HCl (4 mg thrice daily).
   - Azatidine maleate.
6. Piperazine—Hydroxyzine hydrochloride (10 mg or 25 mg thrice daily).

Mechanisms of actions: The main effects are as follows:

1. Anti-cholinergic activity.
2. Anti-inflammatory effect.
3. Anti-allergic effect.
4. Antimotion sickness effects.
5. Anti-emetic activity.
6. Inhibit most responses of smooth muscle to histamine.

Side-Effects

1. *Neurological side-effects*—Sedation, dizziness and tinnitus, blurred vision and diplopia, insomnia, reduced or distributed concentration, irritability and tremors.
2. *Gastrointestinal side-effects*—Anorexia, nausea, vomiting, epigastric distress constipa-

tion (can be minimized by giving them along with food).

3. *Anticholinergic side-effects*—Dry mucous membranes, difficulty in micturition and urinary retention effects, frequency and dysuria, impotence.
4. *Cutaneous side-effects*—Eczematous dermatitis, fixed drug eruption, photosensitivity, urticaria, petechiae.

Class II: Second generation H_1 antihistamines.

They are non-competitive blockers and dissociate slowly from the receptors and have a longer duration of action. They are devoid of sedative and anticholinergic effects these drugs are: acrivastine, astemizole, azelastine, cetrizine, ebastine, fexofenadine, ketotifen, loratidine, mizolastine, terfenadine.

The drugs commonly used are cetirizine (10 mg/day), loratidine (10 mg/day), terfenadine (60 mg BD) and astemizole (10 mg/day), with a loading dose of 10 mg tds × 3 days).

Class III: H_2 anti-histamines—Cimetidine, ranitidine, famotidine, nizatidine.

Class IV: Other drugs with anti-histamine activity—Tricyclic anti-depressants (doxepin), ketotifen, oxafomide.

Indications

1. **Urticaria and angioedema:** Both traditional and second generation antihistamines are found to be useful. The combination of both H_1 and H_2 anti-histamines are very effective in the treatment of acute or chronic idiopathic urticaria and physical urticaries.
2. **Pruritus of various causes:** Viz. dermatitis, papulosquamous disorders, insect bites, etc.
3. **Mast cell disorders:** Ketotifen, cimetidine, azalastine and chlorpheniramine are very effective.
4. **Pruritus due to:** Myelofibrosis, polycythemia and carcinoid flush. Cimetidine is also effective.
5. **The immunodulatory effects** of H_2 antihistamines may offer great therapeutic potential.

Dapsone

Dapsone is a 4,4'—Diaminodiphenyl sulphone. It is weakly bactericidal against M. leprae. It acts by inhibiting folate metabolism in M. leprae. In addition to its anti-bacterial action, it also has anti-inflammatory activity—lysosomal enzymes, interferes with myeloperoxidase system. During daily treatment with 100 mg dapsone, it inhibits the generation of 5-lipoxygenase product in neutrophils.

Dosage

Dose is 6 to 10 mg/kg body weight/week. The average adult dosage is 100 mg/day. For children of 10 to 14 years, it is 50 mg/day of 6 to 9 years it is 25 mg/day.

Indications

Other than its antileprosy action, it is used in dermatology in pemphigus, bullous pemphigoid, dermatitis herpetiformis, subcorneal pustular dermatosis, acne conglobata, systemic lupus erythematosus, vasculitis, lichen planus etc.

Side-Effects

1. Hemolytic anemia especially in G6PD deficient individuals.
2. Agranulocytosis.
3. Hepatitis.
4. Allergic rashes including FDE and exfoliative dermatitis.
5. Dapsone syndrome (fever, jaundice, lymphadenopathy, hepatomegaly and exfoliative dermatitis).
6. Psychosis.

Clofazimine

Clofazimine is a riminophenazien dye. Like dapsone, it is also weakly bactericidal against M.

leprae and virtually monotoxic in the usual dosage used. Clofazimine has both antibacterial and anti-inflammatory activities.

Indications

Apart from its use in multi-drug therapy in leprosy, it is used in dermatology for dermatoses (acne, pustular psoriasis), rhinoscleroma, leishmaniasis, etc.

Dosage

The recommended dose is 50 mg daily.

Side-Effects

1. Reversible dose related reddish to brownish black discolouration of sweat, hair, sputum, urine and faeces.
2. Icthyosis.
3. Phototoxicity, nonspecific skin rashes and anceiform eruptions.
4. Eosinophilic enteropathy.
5. Conjunctival pigmentation.

Methotrexate

Methotrexate (MTX) is a folic acid antagonist and is widely used for the treatment of severe psoriasis.

Dosage

1. Weekly single oral or parental dosage schedule.
2. Intermittent oral schedule of three divided doses 12th hourly over a period of 36 hours each week.
3. Oral dose is 0.4 to 0.6 mg/kg body weight/ week (maximum 30 mg).
4. Parental dose is 15-25 mg/week.

Side-Effects

1. *Gastrointestinal*—Nausea, vomiting, stomatitis, diarrhoea, ulceration, etc.
2. *Hepatitic*—Abnormal liver enzymes, hepatitis, fibrosis and cirrhosis.
3. *Hematopoietic*—Anemia, thrombocytopenia, leucopenia, pancytopenia.
4. *Pulmonary*—Acute hypersensitivity, fibrosis, pneumonia.

Most common side-effect is nausea and vomiting. Serious late side-effect is **cirrhosis of the liver.**

Psoralens

Of the many psoralens isolated and synthesized, three are in routine clinical use. These include 8 methoxypsoralen (8 MOP), 5 methoxypsoralen (5 MOP) and trimethyl psoralen (TMP). They are active only when combined with UVA irradiation. If interferes effects and immunosuppressive effects along with induction of epidermal thickening and melanogenesis.

Dosage

Oral 8 MOP is given in a dose of 0.6 to 0.8 mg/ kg weight/day. Two hours later, the patient is exposed to ultraviolet radiation. A (UVA) at a dose 1 joule/square cm to begin with which is gradually increased to minimal erythema dose depending on the skin type. Therapy is usually given two to three times per week. The number of exposures required for achieving control are usually 15 and 25. Maintenance therapy involves less frequent treatments often as little as once every two to four weeks, with eventual discontinuation of treatment.

Indications

1. Psoriasis.
2. Vitiligo.
3. Photodermatoses.
4. Cutaneous T-cell lymphomas.

Side-Effects

1. Nausea, vomiting.

2. Cutaenous—Acute sunburn and erythema, irreversible hyperpigmentation of the skin, PUVA lentigines, actinic keratoses, premature ageing of the skin.
3. Ocular—Cataract. It can be prevented by using sunglasses on the day of treatment.
4. Carcinogenesis.

Other than oral PUVA therapy, psoralen may be used for topical PUVA therapy and bath PUVA therapy.

Retinoids

Retinoids is a generic term that includes both naturally occurring molecules and also synthetic compounds showing specific biological activities resembling those of vitamin A (retinal).

Synthetic retinoids are produced by chemical modification of vitamin A. Three generations are known today (nonaromatic, monoaromatic and polyaromatic).

First generation (Nonaromatic) includes retinal and compounds that can be derived from it metabolically e.g. retinyl palmitate (topical), retinyl aldehyde (topical), tretinoin (all trans retinoid acid) (topical), 9-cis-retinoic acid, a 14-hydroxyretroretinol, fenretinide (N-[4-hydroxyphenyl]-retinamide), E 5166 (polyprenoic acid).

Second generation (Monoaromatic) by addition of an aromatic ring e.g. etretinate isotretinoin, acitretin, isoacitretin (13-cis-acitretin), motretinide.

Third generation (Arotinoids) e.g. temarotene, arotenoid acid, arotenoid ethylester, arotenoid ethyl sulphone, arotenoid methyl sulphone, adapalene (topical antiance agent), tazarotene (topical antipsoriatic agent).

Intracellularly retinoids interact with cytosolic proteins and then enter the nucleus. By changing the expression of growth factors, ontogenesis, keratin or transglutaminases, retinoids could exert widespread changes in growth and differentiation

Indications of systemic retinoids:

1. Psoriasis and related disorders.
2. Other disorders of keratinization.
3. Seborrhoea, acne and acneiform dermatoses.
4. Rosacea and other acne related dermatoses.
5. Cancers—basal cell carcinoma, actinic keratosis, cutaneous T-cell lymphomas, HIV related Kaposi's sarcoma.
6. Other dermatoses such as lichen planus, lupus erythematosus, lichen sclerosus et atrophicus, prurigo nodularis, photoageing and ageing, pigmentary disorders, etc.

Side-effects of systemic retinoids: The adverse effect profile closely resembles those of hypervitaminosis A. Acute toxicity is dose dependent and reversible.

1. Cheilitis appears 2-3 weeks after initiation of therapy in 100% of patients and is regarded as a marker of sufficient absorption. Other mucocutaneous adverse effects are skin and mucosal dryness, skin fragility and/or stickiness, retinoid dermatitis, palmoplantar desquamation, pruritus, hair loss, paronychia, and photosensitivity.
2. Eye symptomatology and pseudotumor cerebri.
3. Serum lipids and liver function abnormalities.

Chronic Toxicity

1. Bone changes includes hyperostosis, peristosis, osteoporosis, thinning of the bones, premature closure of epiphyses, DISH (diffuse idiopathic skeletal hyperostosis), extraspinal calcification, bone pain and acute arthritis.
2. Arthralgia and myalgias.

Teratogenecity involving central nervous system, skeletal system, cardiovascular system, and other organs.

MULTIPLE CHOICE QUESTIONS

1. The following are correct statements concerning steroids used topically:
A. Halogenation decreases topical activity
B. Thinning of epidermis may occur
C. Thinning of dermis may occur
D. Systemic side-effects commonly occur
E. The rate of epidermal turnover is increased

2. Tacrolimus belongs to which group of drugs?
A. Macrolides
B. Retinoids
C. Anti-cancer drugs
D. Newer penicillins

3. Following are keratolytic agents, *except*:
A. Urea B. Benzoic acid
C. Resorcin D. Salicylic acid

4. The following agents act as sunscreens:
A. PABA
B. Zinc oxide
C. Calamine lotion
D. All of the above

5. Common agent in Lasser's paste and Unna's paste:
A. Zinc oxide B. Gelatin
C. Starch D. Glycerin

6. Zinc is used in the treatment of:
A. Acrodermatitis enteropathica
B. Acne vulgaris
C. Chronic leg ulcers
D. All of the above

7. Among following most potent topical steroid is:
A. Hydrocortisone
B. Clobetasol butyrate
C. Clobetasol propionate
D. Prednisolone

8. Chemicals like monebenzyle ether of hydroquinone cause skin depigmentation by:
A. Inhibiting tyrosinase
B. Destroying melanocytes
C. Preventing transfer of melonosomes
D. Decreasing melanin synthesis

9. The optimum duration of treatment for an effective response with topical minoxidil in male-type alopecia is:
A. 2-4 weeks B. 2-3 months
C. 3-6 months D. 6-12 months

10. The most common side-effect of podofilax gel is:
A. Bleeding B. Itching
C. Pain D. Burning

11. The most frequent side-effect of isotretinoin is:
A. Chest pain B. Cheilitis
C. Arthralgia D. Dizziness

12. Azelaic acid cream is used in the treatment of:
A. Lupus vulgaris
B. DLE
C. Acne vulgaris
D. Psoriasis

1 B,C 2 A 3 B 4 D 5 A 6 D 7 C 8 B 9 D 10 D 11 B
12 C

13. Treatment of tinea veriscolor:

A. Clotrimazole
B. Sodium sulphite
C. Selenium sulphide
D. Miconazole
E. All of the above

14. Hydroquinone compounds cause depigmentation by their action on:

A. Melanocytes
B. Tyrosinase
C. DOPA
D. Melanin

15. All the following are physical sunscreens *except*:

A. Titanium dioxide
B. Zinc oxide
C. Cinnamic acid
D. Calamine

13 E 14 B 15 C

Chapter 24

Recent Advances in Dermatology

LASERS

Different types of laser specific for vascular lesions

Laser type	*Laser characteristics*
Frequency doubled Nd: YAG	532 nm, Q-switched
KTP	532 nm, quasi CW
Krypton	568 nm, quasi CW
Argon-pumped tunable dye	577 nm, quasi CW
Copper vapour	578 nm, quasi CW
Flashlamp-pumped pulsed dye	585 mn, pulsed
Long-pulsed dye	585, 590, 595, 600 nm, pulsed

Noninfectious neutrophilic dermatoses

Nonangiocentric
- Psoriasis
- Reiter's syndrome
- Subcorneal pustular dermatosis
- Acne fulminans
- Blastomycosis-like pyoderma (pyoderma vegetans)
- Neutrophilic eccrine hidradenitis

Angiocentric
- Vessel wall destruction
- Leukocytoclastic vasculitis
- Polyarteritis nodosa

No vessel wall destruction
- Acute febrile neutrophilic dermatosis (Sweet's syndrome)
- Typical
- Atypical

Pyoderma gangrenosum
- Typical
- Atypical

Contd...

Contd...

"Pustular vasculius"
Behcet's disease
Bowel-associated dermatosis-arthritis syndrome
Rheumatoid neutrophilic dermatosis
Pyostomatitis vegetans
Pustular eruption of ulcerative colitis

Familial Mediterranean Fever

Acute febrile neutrophilic dennatosis (Sweet's syndrome): Associated diseases and phenomena

Myetoproliferative disorders
- Myelodysplasia (agnogenic myeloid metaplasia)
- Acute myelocytic leukemia

Hematologic disorders
- Acute myelogenous leukemia
- Chronic myelogenous leukemia
- Myelodysplasia
- Multiple myeloma

Other malignancies (variety of individual reports)
Sarcoidosis
Inflammatory bowel disease
- Crohn's disease
- Ulcerative colitis

Rheumatoid arthritis
Lupus erythematosus
Immunizations
Pregnancy
Postinfectious—bacterial, fungal, parasitic
Behcet's disease
Drug induced
Administration of leukocyte colony—stimulating factors
Hashimoto's thyroiditis

Chapter 25

Metabolic and Nutritional Disorders

PORPHYRIA

- The term "porphyria" is derived from the Greek word for "purple" and originally referred to the red to purple colour of patients affected by acute intermittent porphyria. Other forms of porphyria produce urine that varies from pink to red to brown **(Hersch Test).**
- Porphyrins also account for the fluorescence of urine viewed with a Wood's lamp.
- Almost **all are inherited in an autosomal dominant** pattern except **congenital erythropoietic porphyria which is inherited as autosomal recessive manner.**
- In addition, although the enzyme defects are genetic and permanent, the symptoms are often intermittent and do not appear until puberty except in congenital erythropoietic porphyria and hepatoerythropoietic porphyria (both manifest in infancy or childhood, resemble clinically each other).
- Factors which precipitate are forum's medication, malnutrition and medical illness.

Clinical Classification

- These disorders can be classified into those without vesicobullous lesions and those associated with them.
- The former includes delta aminolevulinic dehydratase deficiency porphyria and acute intermittent porphyria (have no cutaneous manifestations), and erythropoietic protoporphyria (can cause photosensitivity, but vesicobullous lesions are rare).
- The latter includes congenital erythropoietic porphyria (Gunther's disease), hepatoerythropoietic porphyria, hereditary coproporphyria, variegate porphyria (most prevalent in white population of South Africa) and porphyria cutaneous tarda (PCT).

Congenital Erythropoietic Porphyria

- Congenital erythropoietic prophyria manifests in infancy or early childhood.
- It is the result of defective activity of the enzymes uroporphyrinogen cosynthase.
- Clinical manifestations include severe **bullous cutaneous photosensitivity, hypertrichosis, erythrodontia, hemolytic anemia with splenomegaly, and bone abnormalities**. However, the first clue to the diagnosis in infancy is generally not one of these striking cutaneous changes, but **rather the pink or burgundy discoloration of urine.**
- Treatment of this disorder is aimed at the cutaneous photosensitivity or at the anemia and its complications. Sun protection and ingestion of beta carotene may ameliorate some portion of the photodamage. Other modalities, chronic transfusions regimens and splenectomy, the risks must be weighed against the severity of the disorder in each individual case.

PCT

PCT was first recognized by Waldenstrom in the 1930s, who identified a group of patient with excessive porphyrins in the urine, skin lesions in light exposed areas and a late ('tarda') onest in adulthood (in contrast with Gunther's disease), so he called the disease 'porphyria cutanea tarda:

- Clinical signs include darkening of **the urine and cutaneous photosensitivity manifested as fragility and bullae of sun exposed skin, scarring, hypertrichosis and pigmentary and sclerodermoid changes. In severe cases, the clinical appearance may be similar to that of congenital erythropoietic porphyria.**
- Unlike other porphyrias, it is usually not inherited and responds to different treatments (venesection and antimalarias).

Primary Cutaneous Amyloidosis

- Primary cutaneous amyloidosis is defined as cutaneous amyloidosis in the absence of other systemic or dermatological disease.
- The various localized forms of primary cutaneous amyloidosis include the more common papular (lichen amyloidosus) and macular and macular types and the rare nodular or tumefactive form.
- Lichen amyloidosis is the most common form characterized by numerous pruritic, brownish lichenoid papules distributed over the extensor surface of legs and forearms and upper back.
- Macular amyloidosis typically manifests as brownish patches with a reticulate or rippled pattern, involving the upper back, arms and lower extremities.
- In some patients features of both lichen and macular amyloidosis can coexist and the term 'biphasic amyloidosis', has been coined for these. Extensive variants of both macular and popular amyloidosis have also been described.
- On the other hand, amyloidosis cutis dyschromica (ACD) is a rare distinct type of primary cutaneous amyloidosis, which is characterized by reticulate hyperpigmentation with hypopigmented spots seen almost all over the body without any population.
- Treatment is symptomatic with topical corticosteroids and sometimes dermabrasion.

Xanthomatoses

- Xanthomas are composed of masses of lipid containing histocytes forming popular, nodular, and plaque like lesions in the skin, tendons and sometimes in the internal organs. Xanthomas are important clinical findings as they often evolve in the presence of elevated blood lipids and lipoproteins. Lipoproteins are macromolecular complexes that carry hydrophobic plasma lipids, particularly cholesterol and triglycerides, in the plasma. An elevation of serum lipid levels is called hyperlipidemia, or hyperlipoproteinemia while the term dyslipoproteinemia signifies abnormalities in serum lipoproteins, whether or not serum lipid levels are categorically elevated or not. Of clinical interest is the fact that different species of lipoproteins typically different of xanthomas. Thus, the type of xanthoma observed in a particular patient provides important as to the type of hyperlipoproteinemia.

Xanthelasma Palpebraum

- Soft, velvetty papules and plaques arranged around eyelids.
- Common sites—upper eyelid, inner canthus.
- Signify a systemic hyperlipidermia—usually LDL elevations.
- Usually occur in normolipidaemic individuals but may be seen in familial hypercholesterolemia, dysbetalipoproteinemia, mixed hyperlipidermia.

Tuberous Xanthoma

- Firm, yellow—Orange, often with an erythematous halo, small papules (0.5 cm in diameter) to lobulated tumours (2.5 cm or more).
- Usually painless but may be tender on pressure.
- Sites—Knees, elbows, buttocks and pressure points, typically bilateral.
- Seen with raised LDL levels—Familial hypercholesterolemia, dysbetalipoproteinemia and secondary hyperlipidemias (hypothyroidism, chronic biliary disease).

Tendinous Xanthoma

- Slowly enlarging subcutaneous nodules attached to tendons, ligaments, fascia and periosteum (sub-periosteal).
- Overlying skin appears normal.
- Sites—Extensor tendons of hands and feet, Achilles tendon, sub-periosteal bony prominences such as malleoli and elbows.
- Occur in severe hypercholesterolemia in secondary hypercholesterolemia (cholestasis).

Eruptive Xanthoma

- Pinhead sized asymptomatic yellow papules with a reddish, base, usually fleeting in nature and appear in crops.
- Sites—Buttocks, shoulders and extensor surface of extremities.
- Occasionally these papules may coalesce and overlie a tuberous xanthoma—tuberoeruptive xanthomas.
- Associated with pure of mixed hypertriglyceridemia and a high concentration of VLDL or chylmicroma.
- May occur in secondary hyperlipidermia of diabetes mellitus.

Plane Xanthoma

- Yellow—Orange macules or slightly palpable plaques.
- May occur at any site.
- Plane xanthomas over palmar creases—'xanthoma palmaris et striata'—pathognomonic of type III dysbetalipoproteinemia.
- Plane xanthomas may occur in secondary hyperlipidemias (biliary cirrhosis, cholestasis, gammopathy).

Intertriginous Xanthomas

- They appear as flat to slightly yellow dermal plaques with corrugated surface within or adjacent webs, axillae buttocks and antecubital and popliteal fossa.
- They are pathognomonic of type II hypercholestrolemia.

Generalized Plane Xanthomas

- These cover larger areas of the face, neck and thorax and also may involve flexures and palms.
- May be associated with myeloma, macroglobulinemia or lymphoma rarely with normal plasma lipids.
- 50% of patients may have hypolipidemia with low LDL levels.

Cerebrotendinous Xanthomas

- Rare autosomal recessive disorder with xanthomas in the tendons and the brain.
- Defective conversion of cholesterol to bile acids with accumulation of cholesterol.
- Severe neurologic disease and tendency to coronary artery disease.
- Tendon xanthomas.
- Treated with oral deoxycholic acid to replace the bile acid pool (Table 25.1).

Lipoid Proteinosis

- Lipoid proteinosis is a rare disorder characterized by infiltrate of hyaline material into the skin, oral cavity and internal organs.
- It is inherited as a monogenetic autosomal recessive disorder of normal chromosomal pattern.

Table 25.1: Abnormalities of lipoprotein metabolism with their cutaneous features

Lipid phenotype	*Lipoprotein phenotype (Friedrickson)*	*Cutaneous features*
Isolated Hypercholesterolemia		
Familial hypercholesterolemia	IIa	Tuberous xanthomas Tendon xanthomas Subperiosteal xanthomas
Familial defective apo B100	IIa	Tendon xanthomas
Polygenic hypercholesterolemia	IIa	Usually none
Isolated Hypertriglyceridemia		
Familial hypertriglyceridemia	I, V	None, occasionally eruptive xanthoma
Familial lipoprotein lipase deficiency	I, V	Eruptive xanthomas plaques
Familial apo CII deficiency	I, V	Eruptive xanthomas plaques
Hypertriglyceridemia and Hypercholesterolemia		
Combined hyperlipidemia	IIb	Usually none
Dysbetalipoproteinemia	III	Tuberous xanthomas Tuberoeruptive xanthomas Xanthomas striata palmaris

- The earliest manifestation is hoarseness that develops in infancy, which can progress to complete aphonia without breathing difficulty. Examination of larynx frequently reveals infiltration, thickening and nodularity of cords. The mucosa of lip, pharynx and tongue may also develop firm yellow nodules giving it a cobblestone appearance. The tongue and firm on palpation with decreased range of movements. Ankyloglossia can occur due to involvement of the lingual frenulum.
- Deposition of hyaline material along the eyelid margins results in typical beaded papules– 'moniliform blepharosis'. This eyelid is the single most typical clinical feature of this disease. In later stages, there may be total loss of eyelashes. Further infiltration of eyelids leads to its malfunction and can cause corneal ulcer
- Neurological abnormalities include calcification in the hippocampus and falxcerebri and temporal lobe epilepsy.
- The nature of hyaline material and underlying metabolic defect is unknown. It may represent an underlying lysosomal storage disorder with single or multiple enzyme defects, others have postulated it to be a disorder of collagen metabolism or collagen synthesis.
- There is presently no effective therapy for lipoid proteinosis. Hoarseness may be relieved temporarily by surgical removal of vocal cord infiltrates. Facial lesions may be treated by dermabrasion, chemical skin peeling and blepharoplasty. Treatment by oral dimethyl sulphoxide has been claimed to be successful.

Pellagra

- Pellagra is a nutritional disorder that occurs due to niacin deficiency. The term pellagra is derived from the Italian words 'pelle agra' meaning rough skin.
- It is still endemic in areas of Africa and Asia due to poor nutrition and intake of certain cereals such as a maize and jowar (Indian millet) as staple diet.
- In the present day context, in Western world, pellagra is confined to individuals who have

improper food intake such as psychiatry patients, alcoholics and recluses.

- Pellagra is a clinical syndrome characterized by (1) Symmetrical photosensitive skin eruption (2) Gastrointestinal manifestations (3) Neurological and psychiatric disturbances. These well-known group of symptoms are traditionally remembered as pellagra's four D's—dermatitis, diarrhea, dementia and when untreated, death—is very seldom seen. But most of the manifestations are borderline and/or less typical in nature.
- The initial manifestation is an erythematous, photosensitive pruritic rash that occurs on the dorsa of hands.
- The usual sites affected are the face, neck and dorsal surfaces of hands, arms and feet.
- The dorsa of the hands are the most frequent site from where it may extend upward to form the 'glove' or 'gauntlet' of pellagra. The dermatosis is strikingly symmetrical and clearly demarcated from the normal skin.
- The feet is commonly involved and it may also affect the front and back of the leg to form a boot.
- In the face, an erythematous rash extending from the nose to the cheeks, chins, lips, may resemble lupus erythematosus "Butterfly rash". Rarely eyelids and ears may be affected. Facial rash usually occurs concurrently with lesions elsewhere.
- This eruption forms a broadband or collar around the neck, known as Casal's 'necklace'. In many instances, the necklace has an anterior continuation, also known as 'Cravat'.

Aribofalvinosis (Oro-oculo-genital Syndrome)

- This syndrome occurs due to vitamin B_2 (Riboflavin) deficiency and is characterized by mucocutaneous lesions of angular stomatitis, cheilosis, glossitis, seborrhoeic dermatitis (especially around the nose), scrotal and vulvar dermatitis and increased corneal vascularity.
- It usually responds prompty and dramatically to riboflavin supplementation with 5 to 10 mg of riboflavin daily.

Acrodermatitis Enteropathica

- Acrodermatitis enteropathica, an autosomal recessive disorder which appears to be due to defective absorption of zinc from the gastrointestinal tract.
- It may be a presenting sign in cystic fibrosis or AIDS.
- It manifests insidiously between the ages three weeks and 18 months (often when the baby is switched from breast milk to cow's milk) with periorificial (mouth, nose, eyes, ears and perineum) and acral (extensor surfaces of the major joints, fingers and toes) dermatitis, alopecia and diarrhoea (Mnemonic DAD to remember its clinical features.
- The primary cutaneous eruption is vesicobullous, which is symmetrical and grouped. The lesions soon evolve into erosive vesicobullous eruption or psoriasiform patches.
- At the same time or shortly afterward, loss of hair and gastrointestinal disturbances manifested chiefly by diarrhoea, occur.
- Mental depression, listlessness, loss of appetite, perleche and blepharitis may occur during exacerbations.

Laboratory verification of deficient plasma or serum zinc levels may be undertaken where facilities exist, otherwise, all these cases respond to zinc sulphate/gluconate (1 to 2 mg/kg body weight/day) given once or twice daily.

MULTIPLE CHOICE QUESTIONS

1. **Pherynoderma is caused by deficiency of:**
   A. Essential fatty acids
   B. Vitamin A
   C. Vitamin D
   D. Vitamin E
2. **Blue diaper syndrome is due to defect in metabolism of:**
   A. Lysine B. Phenylalanine
   C. Tyrosine D. Tryptophan
3. **Xanthelasma is commonly seen in:**
   A. Hypertension
   B. Diabetes mellitus
   C. Heart failure
   D. Vitamin A deficiency
4. **What is the wavelength of light responsible for sensitivity in poryphyria?**
   A. 220-290 nm B. 290-340 nm
   C. 430-490 nm D. All of the above
5. **Porphyria cutanea tarda can be treated by:**
   A. Phlebotomy
   B. Heme
   C. Low dose chloroquine
   D. Metronidazole
6. **Ocular hallmark of pseudoxanthoma elasticum is:**
   A. Retinal hemorrhage
   B. Iritis
   C. Angoid streak
   D. Keratitis
7. **Hypercholesterolemia is seen in:**
   A. Xanthelasma
   B. Tuberous Xanthoma
   C. Xanthopsia
   D. None of the above
8. **Following are common causes of burning tongue *except:***
   A. Pellagra
   B. Neurosis
   C. Overindulgence in smoking
   D. Ariboflavinosis
9. **Necrobiosis lipoidica diabeticorum is most marked on:**
   A. Forearms B. Face
   C. Front of legs D. Back of legs
10. **Xanthelasma is least common on:**
    A. Upper eyelids B. Lower eyelids
    C. Inner canthus D. None of the above
11. **Which of the following does not cause cutaneous lesion?**
    A. Porphyria cutaneous tarda
    B. Acute intermittent porphyria
    C. Porphyria variegata
    D. Protoporphyria
12. **'Cassals necklace' is a feature of:**
    A. Acrodermatitis enteropathica
    B. Niacin deficiency
    C. Ceruloplasmin deficiency
    D. Essential fatty acid toxicity
13. **Beaded margins of eyelids is a characteristic feature of:**
    A. Granuloma annulare
    B. Leprosy
    C. Erythema annulare centrifugum
    D. Lipoid proteiniosis

1 B 2 D 3 B 4 B 5 C 6 C 7 B 8 D 9 C 10 B 11 B
12 B 13 D

TEST PAPER-2006 (AIPG, AIIMS, UPSC)

1. Which of the following statements about lepromin test is not true?
- **A.** It is negative in most children in first 6 months of life
- **B.** It is a diagnostic test
- **C.** It is an important aid to classify type of leprosy disease
- **D.** It is positive in BB Hansens

2. Anagen phase of the hair indicates:
- **A.** The phase of activity and growth
- **B.** The phase of transition
- **C.** The phase of resting
- **D.** The phase of degeneration

3. 'Chancre redux' is a clinical feature of:
- **A.** Early relapsing syphilis
- **B.** Late syphilis
- **C.** Chancroid
- **D.** Recurrent herpes simplex infection

4. Max Joseph's space is a histopathological feature of:
- **A.** Psoriasis vulgaris
- **B.** Lichen planus
- **C.** Pityriasis rosea
- **D.** Parapsoriasis

5. Ivermectin is indicated in the treatment of:
- **A.** Syphilis
- **B.** Scabies
- **C.** Tuberculosis
- **D.** Dermatophytosis

6. The main cytokine, involved in erythema nodosum leprosum (ENL) reaction, is:
- **A.** Interleukin-2
- **B.** Interferon-gamma
- **C.** Tumor necrosis factor-alpha
- **D.** Macrophage colony stimulating factor

7. The following drug is not used for the treatment of type II lepra reaction:
- **A.** Chloroquin
- **B.** Thalidomide
- **C.** Cyclosporine
- **D.** Corticosteroids

8. The following test is not used for diagnosis of leprosy:
- **A.** Lepromin test
- **B.** Slit skin smear
- **C.** Fine needle aspiration cytology
- **D.** Skin biopsy

9. Air-borne contact dermatitis can be diagnosed by:
- **A.** Skin biopsy
- **B.** Patch test
- **C.** Prick test
- **D.** Estimation of serum IgE levels

10. A patient with HIV disease is on Highly Active Anti-Retroviral Therapy (HAART). He develops tuberculosis. Which one of the following antitubercular drugs interferes with HAART?
- **A.** Isoniazid
- **B.** Ethambutol
- **C.** Pyrazinamide
- **D.** Rifampicin

1 B 2 A 3 A 4 B 5 B 6 C 7 C 8 B 9 B 10 D

11. Which one of the following is the drug of choice for treating systemic fungal infection?

A. Griseofulvin
B. Amphotericin B
C. Ketoconazole
D. Co-trimoxazole

12. A 35-year-old alcoholic presents with diarrhoea and scaly rash on his neck, hands and feet. He will improve if he is treated with which one of the following?

A. Vitamin A
B. Thiamine
C. Folic acid
D. Nicotinic acid

13. Consider the following regarding amelanotic melanoma:

1. **Non-pigmented and appearing as ink or flesh coloured**
2. **Characterized by a radial growth phase**
3. **Inability of these poorly differentiated cancer cells to synthesize melanin pigment**
4. **Precursor lesion is usually lentigo maligna**

Which of the above are correct regarding amelanotic melanoma?

A. 1, 2, 3 and 4 B. 2, 3 and 4 only
C. 1, 3 and 4 only D. 1, 2 and 3 only

14. Which one of the following pairs is not correctly matched ?

A. Acantholysis : P. vulgaris
B. Hypopigmented : Leprosy anaesthetic patch
C. Vesiculobullous : Secondary syphilis lesions
D. Kaposi's Sarcoma : AIDS

15. What is the cutaneous viral infection which is commonly seen in children and characterized by single or multiple pearly-white skin coloured smooth dome shaped papules with central pitting?

A. Chicken pox
B. Small pox
C. Molluscum contagiosum
D. Verruca vulgaris

16. Wegener's Granulomatosis is characterised by the following *except:*

A. Vasculitis of respiratory tract
B. Granulomatous uveitis
C. Granulomatous hepatitis
D. Glomerulonephritis

17. A VDRL reactive mother gave birth to an infant. All of the following would help in determining the risk of transmission to the infant *except:*

A. TPHA test on the serum sample of the mother
B. TPHA test on the serum sample of the infant
C. VDRL on the paired serum sample of the infant and mother
D. Time interval between the treatment of the mother and her delivery

18. A 6-month-old infant had itchy erythematous papules and exudative lesions on the scalp, face, groins and axillae for one month. She also had vesicular lesions on the palms. The most likely diagnosis is:

A. Congenital syphilis
B. Seborrheic dermatitis
C. Scabies
D. Psoriasis

11 B 12 D 13 C 14 C 15 C 16 C 17 B 18 C

19. Pterygium of nail is characteristically seen in:
A. Lichen planus
B. Psoriasis
C. Tinea unguium
D. Alopecia areata

20. A patient had seven irregular hyperpigmented macules on the trunk and multiple small hyperpigmented macules in the axillae and groins since early childhood. There were no other skin lesions. Which is the most likely investigation to support the diagnosis?
A. Slit lamp examination of eye
B. Measurement of intraocular tension
C. Examination of fundus
D. Retinal artery angiography

21. A 24-year-old unmarried woman has multiple nodular, cystic, pustular and comedonic lesions on face, upper back and shoulders for 2 years. The drug of choice for her treatment would be:
A. Acitretin
B. Isotretinoin
C. Doxycycline
D. Azithromycin

22. A 45-year-old farmer has itchy erythematous papular lesions on face, neck, 'V' area of chest, dorsum of hands and forearms for 3 years. The lesions are more severe in summer and improve by 75% in winter. The most appropriate test to diagnose the condition would be:
A. Skin biopsy
B. Estimation of IgE levels in blood
C. Patch test
D. Intradermal prick test

23. Anticentromere antibodies are most commonly associated with:
A. Diffuse cutaneous systemic sclerosis
B. Mixed connective tissue disease
C. CREST syndrome
D. Polymyositis

24. A 40-year-old woman presented to the gynaecologist with complaints of profuse vaginal discharge. There was no discharge from the cervical os on the speculum examination. The diagnosis of bacterial vaginosis was made based upon all of the following findings on microscopy *except:*
A. Abundance of gram variable coccobacilli
B. Absence of lactobacilli
C. Abundance of polymorphs
D. Presence of clue cells

25. Drug induced lupus can be identified by:
A. Anti-histone antibodies
B. Double stranded DNA antibodies
C. Antinuclear antibodies
D. Anti-SM antibodies

19 A 20 A 21 B 22 C 23 C 24 C 25 A

TEST PAPER

1. The mycelium is:
- **A.** A variant of mycetoma
- **B.** Collection of spores
- **C.** A mass of hyphae
- **D.** A mass of yeast cells
- **E.** None of the above

2. The media used for culturing fungus include:
- **A.** Brain-heart infusion anger
- **B.** Sabouraud's agar plus antibiotics
- **C.** Sabouraud's agar
- **D.** All of the above
- **E.** B and C of the above

3. KOH (potassium hydroxide) is used to prepare fungal smears because it:
- **A.** Breaks the septae of hyphae
- **B.** Dissolve keratin
- **C.** Kills bacterial organism
- **D.** All of the above
- **E.** A and B of the above

4. Which of the following are true statements for dermatophytes?
- **A.** Invade only keratinised layer of skin
- **B.** Invade whole of the epidermis
- **C.** Can involve frequently involved
- **D.** Palms and soles never involved

5. Which of the following are two most common superficial mycoses?
- **A.** Pityriasis versicolor
- **B.** Tinea cruris
- **C.** Tinea manum
- **D.** Tinea barbae
- **E.** Tinea capitis

6. 'Black dot' variety of tinea capitis is caused by:
- **A.** Microporum canis
- **B.** Trichophyton violaceum
- **C.** Trichphyton schoenleini
- **D.** Microsporum audouini
- **E.** None of the above

7. In India, majority of the cases of tinea capitis are caused by:
- **A.** Trichophyton violaceum
- **B.** Microsporum audouini
- **C.** Microsporum canis
- **D.** Trichophyton schoenleini
- **E.** None of the above

8. The following are features of favus:
- **A.** Scutula are seen
- **B.** Caused by trichophyton schoenleini
- **C.** Mousy odour is typical
- **D.** Scarring alopecia may result
- **E.** All of the above

9. Which of the following fungi fluoresce under Wood's light?
- **A.** Microsporum audouini
- **B.** Microsporum canis
- **C.** Trichophyton schoenleini
- **D.** All of the above
- **E.** A and C of the above

10. Which of the following statements are true for griseofulvin?
- **A.** Administered orally
- **B.** Is fungistatic
- **C.** Dose is 10 mg/kg/day
- **D.** All of the above
- **E.** B and C of the above

1 C 2 D 3 B 4 A 5 A 6 B 7 A 8 E 9 A 10 D

11. The following is most commonly involved in onychomycosis:
A. Lateral nail folds B. Nail matrix
C. Nail plate D. Nail bed
E. All of the above

12. The cardinal sign of onychomycosis is:
A. Subungual keratotic debris
B. Pitting of nail plate
C. Thinning of nail plate
D. Disintegration of nail plate
E. None of the above

13. Sporotrichosis is caused by:
A. Rhinosporidium seeberi
B. Cladosporium carrionii
C. Sporothrix schenckii
D. Histoplasma capsulatum
E. Cryptococcus neoformans

14. In the classical presentation of sporotrichosis the lesions are seen as:
A. Grouped lesions
B. Scattered lesions
C. Linear lesions along the lymphatics
D. Annular lesions
E. None of the above

15. 'The triad' of mycetoma includes:
A. Tumefaction
B. Sinus tracts
C. Grains/granules
D. Scar marks
E. Vegetative growths

16. All of the following are known aetiological agents of mycetoma *except:*
A. Madurella mycetomatis
B. Allescheria boydii
C. Cryptococcus neoformans
D. Aspergillus nidulans
E. Curvularia lunata

17. Which of the following are not included in subcutaneous mycoses?
A. Histoplasmosis
B. Sporotrichosis
C. Mycetoma
D. Cryptococcosis
E. Chromoblastomycosis

18. Which of the following diseases are opportunistic fungal infections?
A. Sporotrichosis B. Cryptococcosis
C. Mucormycosis D. All of the above
E. B and C both

19. Which of the following factors predispose to candidiasis?
A. Pregnancy
B. Diabetes mellitus
C. Immunosuppressive drugs
D. All of the above
E. B and C of the above

20. Which of the following diseases are caused by viruses?
A. Herpes zoster
B. Kaposi's varicelliforms eruption
C. Herpes genitalis
D. Erythema infectiosum
E. All of the above

21. The most common viral disease seen is:
A. Measles B. Chickenpox
C. Herpes simplex D. Herpes genitalis
E. Verruca vulgaris

22. Which of the following drugs are effective in the treatment of Herpes simplex?
A. Acyclovir B. Corticosteroids
C. Interferons D. Penicillins
E. None of the above

11 A 12 A 13 C 14 C 15 A,B,C 16 C 17 D 18 E 19 D 19 E 20 E
21 E 22 A

23. Paul-Bunnel test is diagnostic of which of the following viral diseases?
A. Molluscum contagiosum
B. Infectious mononucleosis
C. Herpes zoster
D. Verruca vulgaris
E. All of the above

24. The most common bullous eruption seen in adults in India is:
A. Epidermolysis bullosa
B. Pemphigus vulgaris
C. Pemphigoid
D. Dermatitis herpetiformis
E. None of the above

25. Kaposi's varicelliform eruption is caused by the following viruses:
A. Vaccinia virus
B. Herpes virus
C. Papilloma viruses
D. Coxsackie virus
E. All of the above

26. Molluscum contagiosum is caused by which of the following viruses:
A. Herpes group of viruses
B. Pox group of viruses
C. Coxsackie virus
D. Epstein-Barr viruses
E. All of the above

27. Which of the following features is seen in Herpes zoster?
A. Unilateral involvement
B. Grouped vesicles on normal skin
C. Isolated vesicles on erythematous skin
D. Mucous membranes are involved
E. Incubation period of 7 to 12 days

28. The complications of Herpes zoster include:
A. Scarring
B. Post-herpetic neuralgia
C. Secondary bacterial infection
D. All of the above
E. A and B of the above

29. The following are manifestations of chicken pox:
A. Polymorphic rash
B. Fever
C. Centripetal rash
D. Vesicular rash
E. All of the above

30. The clinical features of verruca vulgaris include:
A. Firm papules
B. Verrucous surface
C. Occur at the site of trauma
D. Asymptomatic
E. All of the above

31. The clinical types of warts incude:
A. Plane warts
B. Filliform warts
C. Plantar warts
D. Verruca vulgaris
E. All of the above

32. The clinical features of condylomata accuminata are:
A. Pinkish papulo-plaques
B. Soft tumour
C. Hard tumour
D. All of the above
E. A and B of the above

33. The following are used in treating warts:
A. Intralesional bleomycin
B. Podophyllin resin
C. 5% Fluorouracil
D. Carbon dioxide laser
E. All of the above

23 B 24 B 25 E 26 B 27 A 28 D 29 E 30 E 31 E 32 E 33 E

34. The following cutaneous lesions are seen in hepatitis B infections:
- A. Erythema nodosum
- B. Morbilliform rash
- C. Urticaria
- D. All of the above
- E. B and C

35. Which of the following causes scabies in man?
- A. Sarcoptes scabiei var. hominis
- B. Sarcoptes scabiei var. canis
- C. Cheyletiella yasguri
- D. Acarus sira
- E. Pediculus humanus

36. The average number of adult female mites in an adult patient of scabies is:
- A. 10-14
- B. 15-50
- C. 50-100
- D. 100-200
- E. More than 20,000

37. The minimum number of mites required to produce scabies is:
- A. One gravid female mite
- B. One female mite
- C. 10 female mites
- D. 20 female mites
- E. 30 female and male mites each

38. The time taken to start itching after acquiring mite for the first time is:
- A. 2 days
- B. 1 weeks
- C. 2 weeks
- D. 8 weeks
- E. 12 weeks

39. The pathognomonic lesion of scabies is:
- A. Papule
- B. Vesicle
- C. Burrow
- D. Nodule
- E. Urticarial papule

40. Clinical manifestations of scabies include the following:
- A. Burrow
- B. Nodular lesions on scrotum
- C. Nocturnal itching
- D. Urticarial papules
- E. All of the above

41. Complications of scabis include the following:
- A. Bacterial infections
- B. Glomerulonephritis
- C. Serum sickness
- D. Sub-acute bacterial endocarditis
- E. None of the above

42. Norwegian scabies is usually seen in the following conditions:
- A. Leukaemia
- B. Prolonged use of immunosuppressive
- C. Mongolism
- D. Diabetes
- E. All of the above

43. All of the following are antiscabetic agents *except*:
- A. Benzyl benzoate
- B. Gammabenzene hexachloride
- C. Crotamiton
- D. Selenium sulfide
- E. Precipitated sulphur

44. Pediculosis is caused by:
- A. Mites
- B. Sucking lice
- C. Ticks
- D. Fleas
- E. None of the above

45. The manifestation of pediculosis capitis includes:
- A. Matting of hair
- B. Itching on the scalp
- C. Secondary bacterial infection
- D. Foul odour
- E. All of the above

34 D 35 A 36 A 37 C 38 D 39 C 40 E 41 A,B 42 E 43 D 44 A 45 E

46. Which of the following are not features of nits?
A. Can be easily picked from hair
B. Can be slided along the hair
C. Are the egg capsules of lice
D. Deposits at the ends of hair
E. All of the above

47. The following medications are used for the treatment of pediculosis capitis:
A. Gammabenzene hexachloride
B. Malathion
C. 5% emulsion of DDT
D. All of the above
E. A and C of the above

48. The manifestations of pediculosis coporis include:
A. Itching
B. Seams of clothes
C. Body hair
D. Genitalia
E. All of the above

49. The pubic louse can be found at which of the following sites?
A. Pubic hair
B. Abdominal hair
C. Thigh hair
D. Axillary hair
E. All of the above

50. Papular urticaria is an acquired sensitivity to mites by:
A. Human fleas
B. Bed bugs
C. Mosquitoes
D. Animal fleas
E. All of the above

51. The following protozoa cause cutaneous leishmaniasis:
A. Leishmania donovani
B. Leishmania tropica
C. Leishmania braziliensis
D. All of the above
E. A and B of the above

52. Clinical manifestations of cutaneous leishmaniasis include:
A. Ulcerated nodules
B. Nodules
C. Plaques
D. Papules in and around scar
E. All of the above

53. Delhi boil/Oriental sore is:
A. A form of cutaneous leishmaniasis
B. A sexually transmitted disease
C. Mycobacterial infections
D. Deep fungal infection
E. None of the above

54. The most common cause of cutaneous larva migrans is:
A. Ancylostoma braziliense
B. Toxocara canis
C. Ascaris lumbricoides
D. Strongyloides stercoralis
E. None of the above

55. The clinical manifestation seen in larva migrans include:
A. Itching
B. Wandering linear eruption
C. Vesicles along the tracts
D. Series of loops and tortuous tracks
E. All of the above

56. The following are features of eczemas:
A. Distinctive patterned inflammation of skin (dermatitis)
B. Caused by external factors
C. Genetically determined
D. All of the above
E. A and C both

46 A 47 D 48 E 49 E 50 E 51 D 52 E 53 B 54 C 55 E 56 D

57. **The following are endogenous eczema *except:***
A. Irritant contact dermatitis
B. Seborrheic dermatitis
C. Pityriasis alba
D. Atopic dermatitis
E. Pompholyx

58. **The exogenous eczemas include:**
A. Infective dermatitis
B. Allergic contact dermatitis
C. Irritant contact dermatitis
D. All of the above
E. B and C both

59. **The manifestations of atopic diathesis include:**
A. Atopic dermatitis
B. Bronchial asthma
C. Hay fever
D. All of the above
E. A and B both

60. **The phases of atopic dermatitis include:**
A. Infantile phase
B. Childhood phase
C. Adult phase
D. All of the above
E. A and B both

61. **The clinical features of seborrhoeic dermatitis include:**
A. Yellowish to erythematous papules
B. Greasy scales
C. Petaloid lesions
D. Follicular lesions
E. All of the above

62. **The clinical features of pityriasis Alba include:**
A. Mainly seen in children
B. Round or oval irregular plaque
C. Fine branny scales
D. Hypopigmentation
E. All of the above

63. **The clinical features of gravitational (stasis) eczema include:**
A. Lower legs commonly invlolved
B. Seen in middle aged
C. Varicosity of superficial veins
D. Diffuse brown pigmentation
E. All of the above

64. **The clinical features of pompholyx include:**
A. Sudden onset
B. Deep seated papulo-vesicles on palms and soles
C. Itching
D. Bullae on palms and soles
E. All of the above

65. **The irritant contact dermatitis include:**
A. Acute irritant dermatitis
B. Irritant reaction
C. Cumulative irritant dermatitis
D. All of the above
E. A and C

66. **The common allergens causing ballergic contact dermatitis in India include:**
A. Chromium salts
B. Nickel
C. Parthenium plants
D. Neomycin
E. All of the above

67. **The most common topical antibiotic causing contact allergic dermatitis is:**
A. Framycetin
B. Neomycetin
C. Nitrofurazone
D. Gentamycin
E. Fusidic acid

57 A 58 D 59 D 60 D 61 E 62 E 63 E 64 E 65 D 66 B 67 A

68. The diagnosis of contact dermatitis is confirmed by:

A. Patch tests
B. Biopsy
C. History of exposure to allergen
D. Clinical feature
E. All of the above

69. The following are useful in the treatment of atopic dermatitis:

A. Topical corticosteroids
B. Coal tar paste
C. Topical corticosteroids under occlusion
D. Photochemotherapy
E. All of the above

70. The following dematoses can have abnormal reactions on exposure to cold:

A. Scleroderma
B. Systemic lupus erythematosus
C. Syphilis
D. Cold urticaria
E. All of the above

71. Decubitus ulcer (bedsore) is caused by which of the following:

A. Prolonged pressure
B. Cold
C. Becterial infection
D. Heat
E. All of the above

72. The following statement are true for corn:

A. Circumscribed lesion
B. Surface is shiny
C. Central hard core
D. Bony spur beneath core
E. All of the above

73. Sun burn is mainly caused by which of the following?

A. UVC
B. UVA
C. UVB
D. Infrared
E. Visible light

74. The correct wavelength of UVB is:

A. 240-290 nm
B. 290-320 nm
C. 320-400 nm
D. 400-700 nm
E. None of the above

75. The dermatitis, which occurs with the use of eau de cologne, is:

A. Eczematous dermatitis
B. Berloque dermatitis
C. Seborrhoeic dermatitis
D. Phytophoto dermatitis
E. Photoallergic dermatitis

76. The following are photosensitive disorders:

A. Xeroderma pigmentosum
B. Pellagra
C. Porphyria
D. Systemic lupus erythematosus
E. All of the above

77. The following disorders have an autosomal dominant inheritance:

A. Neurofibromatosis
B. Ichthyosis vulgaris
C. Tuberous sclerosis
D. Tylosis
E. All of the above

78. The following are features of incontinentia pigment:

A. Distinctive cutaneous lesions
B. Skeletal abnormalities
C. Eye changes
D. Delayed dentition
E. All of the above

68 A 69 E 70 D 71 E 72 E 73 C 74 B 75 B 76 E 77 E 78 E

79. **The "fountain-spray splatters" pigmentation is characterized of which of the following diseases?**
A. Arsenic pigmentation
B. Incontinentia pigment
C. Tuberous sclerosis
D. Xeroderma pigmentosum
E. Phenylketonuria

80. **Phakomatoses include the following:**
A. Congenital retinal tumors
B. Cutaneous involvement
C. CNS involvement
D. All of the above
E. A and B both

81. **Phakomatoses comprises the following disorders:**
A. Tuberous sclerosis
B. Von Recklinghausen's disease
C. Ataxia-telangiectasia
D. Sturge-Weber syndrome
E. All of the above

82. **The following are features of tuberous sclerosis:**
A. Adenoma sebaceum
B. Subungual fibromas
C. Shagreen patch
D. Mental retardation
E. All of the above

83. **Axillary freckling (Crowe's sign) is seen in which of the following diseases?**
A. Ataxia-telangiectasia
B. Neurofibromatosis
C. Peutz-Jeghers syndrome
D. Pinta
E. Leishmaniasis

84. **Following are the features of neurofibromatosis:**
A. Café-au-lait macules
B. Iris lisch nodules
C. Cutaneous neurofibromas
D. Epilepsy
E. All of the above

85. **The following types of ichthyoses have autosomal dominant inheritance:**
A. Ichthvosis vulgaris
B. X-linked ichthyosis
C. Lamellar ichthyosis
D. Episermolytic hyperkeratosis
E. None of the above

86. **The following are features of ichthyosis vulgaris:**
A. Onset at childhood
B. Fine and white scales
C. Corneal opacities
D. Follicular keratotic lesions
E. All of the above

87. **Steroid sulfatase is absent in the following ichthyosis:**
A. Lamellar ichthyosis
B. X-linked ichthyosis
C. Ichthyosis vulgaris
D. All of the above
E. A and C both

88. **The risk of malignant transfusion exists in the following naevi:**
A. Naevus sebaceous
B. Epidermal naevus
C. Congenital melanocytic naevus
D. All of the above
E. A and C both

89. **Pigmented hairy epidermal naevus (Becker's naevus) is:**
A. Melanocytic naevus
B. Vascular naevus
C. Epidermal naevus
D. Sebaceous naevus
E. Connective tissue naevus

79 B 80 D 81 E 82 E 83 B 84 E 85 A 86 E 87 B 88 E 89 A

90. The vascular naevi which gradually disappear with increasing age are:
A. Salmon patch
B. Portwine stain
C. Cavernous haemangiomas
D. All of the above

91. Cavernous-hemangiomas can be complicated by:
A. Malignant change
B. Haemorrhage
C. Ulceration
D. B and C both
E. All of the above

92. Basal cell carcinoma is characterized by:
A. Lesions predominantly over head and neck
B. Rolled out pearly border
C. Ulceration
D. All of the above
E. A and C both

93. The clinical types of basal cell carcinoma are:
A. Rodent ulcer
B. Pearly papulo-nodular
C. Pigmented
D. Morphea like
E. All of the above

94. The diagnosis of basal cell carcinoma is best conformed by:
A. Lymph node biopsy
B. Skin biopsy
C. Cytological examination from the lesion
D. All of the types
E. A and C

95. Squamous cell carcinoma is characterized by:
A. Frequent metastases to regional lymph nodes
B. Spreading non-healing ulcer
C. Cauliflower like growth
D. All of the above
E. A and B

96. The common clinical types of cutaneous malignant melanoma is:
A. Nodular melanoma
B. Lentigo maligna melanoma
C. Superficial spreading melanoma
D. Subungual malignant melanoma
E. All of the above

97. The benign tumors of fibrous tissue include:
A. Dermatofibroma
B. Keloid
C. Hypertrophic scar
D. All of the above
E. B and C both

98. The following are tumours of blood vessels:
A. Granuloma telangiectaticum
B. Glomus tumour
C. Kaposi's sarcoma
D. Lymphangiosarcoma
E. All of the above

99. Common skin disorders seen in infancy include:
A. Mongolian spot
B. Miliaria
C. Seborrheic dermatitis
D. Atopic dermatitis
E. All of the above

100. Common vesiculo-bullous disorder seen in children include:
A. Chronic bullous dermatosis of childhood
B. Epidermolysis bullosa
C. Popular urticaria
D. Bullous impetigo
E. All of the above

90 C 91 D 92 D 93 E 94 D 95 D 96 E 97 D 98 E 99 E 100 E

101. Manifestations of chronic bullous dermatosis of childhood include:
- A. Onset below the age of 5 years
- B. Large tense bullae
- C. Trunk and genitalia involved
- D. Pruritus
- E. All of the above

102. Which of the following are involved in the pathogenesis of napkin dermatosis?
- A. Ammoniacal elements
- B. Maceration due to wet diapers
- C. Prolonged contact with urine and faeces
- D. Contact with irritants
- E. All of the above

103. Napkin dermatitis is secondarily infected with which of the following organisms?
- A. Staphylococcus aureus
- B. Streptococcus pyogenes
- C. Candida albicans
- D. Pseudomonas aerruginosa
- E. None of the above

104. The presence of satellite lesion in napkin dermatitis indicate:
- A. Secondary invasion by candida albicans
- B. Immunodeficiency
- C. Bacterial infection
- D. B and C of the above
- E. All of the above

105. Cradle cap like lesions are seen in which of the following diseases?
- A. Seborrheic dermatitis
- B. Nummular dermatitis
- C. Psoriasis vulgaris
- D. Ichthyosis vulgaris
- E. None of the above

106. The following are clinical features of erythema toxicum neonatorum:
- A. Seen in 50% of term infants
- B. Initial eruption is a blotchy red macule
- C. Commonly appears on trunk
- D. Onset in first 48 hours after birth
- E. All of the above

107. Acrodermatitis enteropathica is due to the deficiency of which of the following?
- A. Iron
- B. Zinc
- C. Copper
- D. Magnesium
- E. None of the above

108. Clinical manifestations of acrodermatitis enteropathica include:
- A. Diarrhoea
- B. Exudative eczematous eruption
- C. Periorificial skin involved
- D. Sparse hair
- E. All of the above

109. Causes of patchy alopecia in children include:
- A. Alopecia aerata
- B. Secondary syphilis
- C. Follicular mucinosis
- D. All of the above
- E. A and B

110. Common birthmarks in infants include:
- A. Portwine stain
- B. Mongolian haemangioma
- C. Cavernous haemongioma
- D. Melanocytic naevus
- E. All of the above

111. The age related changes in the skin include: Dryness .....:
- A. Wrinkling
- B. Sparse and gray hair
- C. Benign skin tumours
- D. All of the above

101 E 102 E 103 C 104 A 105 A 106 E 107 B 108 E 109 D 110 E 111 D

112. The most common benign tumour associated with ageing of skin is:
A. Senile sebaceous hyperplasia
B. Seborrheic keratosis
C. Skin tags
D. Keratoacanthoma
E. Senile angiomata

113. The site at which seborrheic keratosis occurs are:
A. Face B. Palms and soles
C. Trunk D. Limbs
E. All of the above

114. Manifestations of solar elastosis include:
A. Wrinkling
B. Senile purpura
C. Senile comedones
D. Laxity of skin
E. All of the above

115. The important causes of blisters in the elderly include:
A. Pemphigoid
B. Diabetes mellitus
C. Porphyria cutaneous tarda
D. Toxic epidermal necrolysis
E. All of the above

116. Which of the following sites are predominantly involved in acne vulgaris?
A. Face B. Scalp
C. Trunk D. Buttocks
E. All of the above

117. Which of the following factors are involved in the causation of acne?
A. Excess sebum production
B. Alteration in the constituents of sebum
C. Altered androgen oestrogen ratio
D. Propionibacterium acnes
E. All of the above

118. The following cutaneous lesions are seen in acne vulgaris:
A. Comedones
B. Pustules
C. Papules
D. Cysts
E. All of the above

119. The pathognomic lesion of acne is:
A. Comedone B. Pustule
C. Cyst D. Nodule
E. Papule

120. Acneiform eruptions are caused by which of the following drugs?
A. Corticosteroids B. Isoniazid
C. Iodides D. Vitamin B_{12}
E. All of the above

121. Acneiform eruptions differ from classical acne vulgaris by which of the following?
A. Abrupt onset
B. Trunk commonly involved
C. Predominantly popular lesions
D. Clear on withdrawal of offending drug
E. All of the above

122. Which of the following cutaneous lesions are seen in rosacea?
A. Erythema
B. Papule
C. Pustule
D. Telangiectasia
E. All of the above

123. Rhinophyma is a complication of which of the following diseases?
A. Rosacea
B. Progressive systematic sclerosis
C. Urticaria pigmentosa
D. Rhinoscleroma
E. Acne vulgaris

112 B 113 A 114 E 115 A 116 A 117 E 118 E 119 A 120 E 121 E 122 E 123 A

124. The following drugs can cause alopecia:
- A. Methotrexate
- B. Cyclophosphamide
- C. Retinoids
- D. All of the above
- E. A and B both

125. "Patterned alopecia" is the term used for which of the following?
- A. Common male baldness
- B. Common female baldness
- C. Congenital alopecia
- D. Alopecia areata
- E. Pseudopelade

126. Which of the following is false about alopecia areata?
- A. Cicatricial alopecia seen
- B. Exclamation mark hair
- C. Newly lost hair are club hair
- D. Nails involved
- E. Recurrences seen

127. The following are true about telogen effuvium:
- A. Club hairs are shed
- B. Alopecia is diffuse
- C. Seen after acute febrile illness
- D. Hair loss increases spontaneously
- E. All of the above

128. All of the following drugs can cause hypertrichosis *except:*
- A. Chloroquine
- B. Dilantin
- C. Corticosteroids
- D. Minoxidil
- E. Penicillamine

129. All of the following conditions can cause hirsutism *except:*
- A. Addison's disease
- B. Stein-Levanthal syndrome
- C. Ovarian tumours
- D. Acromegaly
- E. Testosterone therapy

130. Generalized hypertrichosis can be seen in the following conditions *except:*
- A. Anorexia nervosa
- B. Porphyria cutanea tarda
- C. Penicillamine
- D. Diabetes mellitus
- E. Juvenile hypothyroidism

131. Miliaria crystalline is seen commonly after:
- A. High grade fever
- B. Sunburn
- C. Application of corticosteroids
- D. After cold bath
- E. All of the above

132. Which of the following is commonly known as "Prickly Heat"?
- A. Miliaria crystalline
- B. Miliaria rubra
- C. Miliaria profounda
- D. Fox-Fordyce diseases
- E. None of the above

133. Fox-Fordyce diseases is a disorder of which of the following structures?
- A. Apocrine glands
- B. Eccrine glands
- C. Sebaceous glands
- D. Hair follicle
- E. None of the above

134. Which of the following are disorders of apocrine glands?
- A. Bromohidrosis
- B. Fox-Fordyce disease
- C. Hidredenitis suppurativa
- D. All of the above
- E. None of the above

124 D 125 A 126 A 127 E 128 A 129 A 130 C 131 A 132 B 133 A 134 B

135. The following are true about hidradenitis suppurativa:
A. Commonly involves axilla
B. Scarring and sinuses seen
C. Anogenital area may be involved
D. All of the above
E. None of the above

136. Urticarial lesions show combinations of:
A. Vascular dilatation
B. Oedema
C. Infilteration of dermis with cells
D. Changes in mast cell granules
E. All of the above

137. The following are known mediators in urticaria:
A. Histamine
B. Leukotrienes (SRS)
C. Prostaglandins
D. Kinins
E. All of the above

138. Anaphylaxis involves which of following types of allergic mechanisms?
A. Type I allergic reaction
B. Type II allergic reaction
C. Type III allergic reaction
D. Type IV allergic reaction
E. All of the above

139. Hereditary angioedema is due to the deficiency of which of the following?
A. Inhibitor of C_1 esterase
B. C_2 esterase
C. IgA
D. IgG
E. All of the above

140. Which of the following inherited conditions can produce urticaria?
A. Familial cold urticaria
B. C_3 inhibitor deficiency
C. Amyloidosis
D. Epidermolysis bullosa dystrophica
E. All of the above

141. Which of the following lesions are seen in cholinergic urticaria?
A. Small 1 to 2 mm sized wheals
B. Large areas of erythema surrounding wheals
C. Giant wheals
D. Swelling of mucous membranes
E. Purpuric lesions

142. Esthema nodosum is predominantly located on:
A. Flexor aspects of lower legs
B. Extensor aspects of lower legs
C. Flexor aspects of upper limbs
D. Extensor aspects of upper limbs
E. Face

143. Recurrent erythema multiforma is commonly associated with:
A. Herpes simplex
B. Amoebiasis
C. Hepatitis-B
D. Mycoplasma pneumoniae
E. All of the above

144. Target (Iris) lesions is characterized of:
A. Erythema nodosum
B. Parapsoriasis
C. Erythema multiforme
D. Pyoderma gangrenosum
E. All of the above

145. Which of the following figurative erythema is associated with internal malignancy?
A. Erythema annulare centrifugum
B. Erythema gyratum repens
C. Erythema marginatum rheumaticum
D. Erythema chronicum migrans
E. All of the above

135 D 136 E 137 E 138 A 139 A 140 B 141 A 142 B 143 A 144 C 145 B

146. Which of the following diseases can be associated with pyoderma gangrenosum?
A. Ulcerative colitis
B. Rheumatoid arthritis
C. Leukaemia
D. Paraproteinaemias
E. All of the above

147. Which of the following are seen in Behcet's disease?
A. Recurrent non-specific urethritis
B. Recurrent apthous ulceration
C. Recurrent genital ulceration
D. Arthritis
E. All of the above

148. The following are features of sweet syndrome:
A. Fever
B. Erythematous, painful plaques
C. Raised ESR
D. Dramatic response to corticosteroids
E. All of the above

149. The correct sequence of events seen in Raynaud's phenomenon is:
A. Rubber, cyanosis and pallor
B. Pallor, rubor and cyanosis
C. Pallor, cyanosis and rubor
D. Cyanosis, rubor and pallor
E. Cyanosis, pallor and rubor

150. The following drugs can cause Raynaud's phenomenon:
A. Ergot B. Propranolol
C. Sulfasalazine D. Arsenic
E. All of the above

151. Which of the following conditions can be associated with Raynaud's phenomenon?
A. Scleroderma
B. Carpal tunnel syndrome
C. Atherosclerosis obliterans
D. Cryoglobulinaemia
E. All of the above

152. Drug induced lupus erythematosus can be caused by which of the following drugs?
A. Griseofulvin B. Procainamide
C. Isoniazid D. Hydralazine
E. All of the above

153. Lichenoid drug eruption can be caused by which of the following?
A. Mepacrine
B. β-blockers
C. Thiazides
D. Chloroquine
E. All of the above

154. Which of the following is the most common cutaneous side effect of griseofulvin?
A. Stevens-Johnson syndrome
B. Morbilliform rash
C. Photodermatitis
D. Gastrointestinal disturbances
E. Lupus erythematosus like rash

155. The beta-blockers drugs can cause the following *except:*
A. Erythroderma
B. Lichenoid eruption
C. Psoriasis
D. Lupus erythematosus like syndrome
E. All of the above

156. Erythroderma is commonly caused by which of the following drug?
A. Chloroquine B. Arsenicals
C. Phenytoin D. Sulfonamide
E. All of the above

146 E 147 E 148 E 149 C 150 A 151 E 152 E 153 E 154 D 155 E 156 E

157. The common drugs causing increased pigmentation are:
A. Chorpromazine B. Phenytoin
C. Arsenic D. Antimalariais
E. All of the above

158. Which of the following drugs can cause alopecia?
A. Retinoids B. Methotrexate
C. Propranolol D. Lithium
E. All of the above

159. Erythema nodosum can be caused by the following drugs *except:*
A. Salicylates B. Glucocorticoids
C. Iodides D. Sulfonamides
E. Tetracycline

160. Which of the following drugs can induce hair color change?
A. Chloroquine
B. Resorcinol
C. Dithranol
D. Hydrogen peroxide
E. All of the above

161. Which of the following drugs can cause hirsutism?
A. Testosterone
B. Anabolic steroids
C. Progesterones
D. All of the above
E. A and C of the above

162. Which of the following drugs can cause hypertrichosis?
A. Diazoxide B. Phenytoin
C. Thiazides D. Allopurinol
E. All of the above

163. Which of the following drugs can cause lymphadenopathy?
A. Carbamazepine B. Phenytoin
C. Phenylbutazone D. Cephaloridine
E. All of the above

164. Which of the following drugs can cause discolouration of nails?
A. Chloroquine
B. Tetracycline
C. Cyclophosphamide
D. Chlorpromazine
E. All of the above

165. Which of the following drugs can cause purpuric lesions?
A. Chlorpropamide
B. Tetracycline
C. Barbiturates
D. Coaltar products
E. All of the above

166. Which of the following drugs can cause toxic epidermal necrolysis?
A. Phenytoin B. Sulfonamides
C. Barbiturates D. Phenylbutazone
E. All of the above

167. Which of the following drugs can exacerbate porphyria?
A. Chloroquine B. Barbiturates
C. Oestrogens D. Griseofulvin
E. All of the above

168. Sulfonamides can cause which of the following cutaneous reactions?
A. Bullous erythema multiforma
B. Exanthems
C. Photosensitivity
D. All of the above
E. A and C of the above

169. Penicillin can cause which of the following cutaneous reactions?
A. Bullous erythema multiforma
B. Serum sickness
C. Vasculitis
D. Anaphylaxis
E. All of the above

157 E **158** E **159** B **160** E **161** D **162** B **163** E **164** E **165** A **166** E **167** E **168** D **169** E

170. Phenytoin can produce which of the following cutaneous reactions?
- A. Morbilliform rash
- B. Erythema multiforme
- C. Exfoliative dermatitis
- D. Pseudolymphoma syndrome
- E. All of the above

171. Gold salts can produce which of the following cutaneous lesions?
- A. Exfoliative dermatitis
- B. Pigmentation
- C. Lichenoid eruption
- D. All of the above

172. The following are useful in managing drug eruptions:
- A. Hospitalization
- B. Careful monitoring
- C. Regular reassessment
- D. Symptomatic treatment
- E. All of the above

173. Which of the following mechanisms may be involved in the pathogenesis of vitiligo?
- A. Autoimmunity
- B. Neurological factors
- C. Autocytotoxicity
- D. Chemical cytotoxicity
- E. All of the above

174. Vitiligo may be associated with which of the following diseases?
- A. Diabetes mellitus
- B. Pernicious anaemia
- C. Thyroid disease
- D. Halo naevus
- E. All of the above

175. Photochemotherapy for vitiligo is best administered:
- A. Daily
- B. Alternate days
- C. Every fifth day
- D. Once a week
- E. None of the above

176. The pigmented macules in Peutz-Jeghers syndrome are most commonly seen on:
- A. Buccal mucosa
- B. Lips
- C. Fingers (Dorsum of hands)
- D. Periorally
- E. All of the above

177. Which of the following drugs may exacerbate psoriasis?
- A. Chloroquine
- B. Lithium
- C. Mepacrine
- D. Psoralens
- E. Methotrexate

178. Which of the following histopathological features are diagnostic of psoriasis?
- A. Munro's microabscesses
- B. Spongiform pustule of Kogoj
- C. Acanthosis
- D. Extensive parakeratosis
- E. All of the above

179. Which of the following morphological features are seen in psoriasis?
- A. Silvery white scales
- B. Commonly seen on limbs and trunk
- C. Well circumscribed lesions
- D. Scaly erythematous papules and plaques
- E. All of the above

170 E 171 D 172 E 173 E 174 E 175 B 176 E 177 A 178 B 179 E

180. Auspitz's sign in psoriasis is taken as positive when:
A. Fine bleeding point seen on scales removal
B. Thin transparent membrane seen on scales removal
C. Easy removal of scales
D. Lesions at the site of trauma
E. Pale skin surrounding the psoriasis plaque

181. Koebner's phenomenon is seen in which of the following diseases?
A. Psoriasis vulgaris
B. Lichen planus
C. Pemiphigus vulgaris
D. Alopecia areata
E. Lupus vulgaris

182. Which of the following is the most common manifestation of psoriasis on nails?
A. Pitting
B. Onycholysis
C. Thickening of nails
D. Discolouration
E. Subungual hyperkeratosis

183. Which of the following joint involvement is the most diagnostic of psoriasis?
A. Proximal interphalangeal
B. Distal interphalangeal joints
C. Metacarpophalangeal joints
D. Knee joints
E. All of the above

184. Pustular psoriasis may be precipitated by which of the following?
A. Nystatin
B. Salicylates
C. Sudden withdrawal of systemic steroids
D. Iodides
E. All of the above

185. The following therapeutic agents can be used for treating psoriasis:
A. Cyclosporine A
B. Methotrexate
C. Topical corticosteroids
D. Topical dithranol
E. All of the above

186. Herald patch is typical of which of the following diseases?
A. Psoriasis
B. Pityriasis rosea
C. Lichen planus
D. Urticaria pigmentosa
E. Erythema multiforme

187. The typical skin lesions seen in pityriasis rosea include:
A. Herald patch
B. Discrete oval erythematous patch with collarette of scales
C. Target lesion
D. Nodular lesions on trunk
E. None of the above

188. The "short contact therapy" in psoriasis can be done with:
A. Dithranol
B. Topical steroids
C. Coaltar
D. Methotrexate
E. Any of the above

189. The classical features of lichen planus include:
A. Polygonal, flat violaceous papules
B. Wickham's striae
C. Koebner's phenomenon
D. Itching
E. All of the above

180 A 181 A,B 182 E 183 B 184 C 185 E 186 B 187 A,B 188 A 189 E

190. Wickham's striae are seen in which of the following diseases?
- **A.** Psoriasis
- **B.** Lichen planus
- **C.** Lichen nitidus
- **D.** Pityriasis rosea
- **E.** All of the above

191. The following nail changes are seen in lichen planus:
- **A.** Thinning of nail
- **B.** Longitudinal grooves
- **C.** Pterygium unguis
- **D.** Onycholysis
- **E.** All of the above

192. The following lesions are characteristic of lichen nitidus:
- **A.** Flaccid bullae
- **B.** Keratotic papules
- **C.** Polygonal violaceous papules
- **D.** Small, smooth, circular minipapules
- **E.** Scaly erythematous plaques

193. Lichen planus may occur as part of:
- **A.** Psoriasis
- **B.** Graft versus host disease
- **C.** Lupus erythematosus
- **D.** All of the above
- **E.** B and C

190 B **191** E **192** D **193** D